Men Who Control Women's Health

Men Who Control Women's Health

The Miseducation of Obstetrician-Gynecologists

Diana Scully

Houghton Mifflin Company Boston 1980

Library of Congress Cataloging in Publication Data

Scully, Diana.
Men who control women's health.

Bibliography: p.
Includes index.
1. Gynecology — Study and teaching (Graduate) — United States. 2. Obstetrics — Study and teaching (Graduate) — United States. 3. Sexism in medicine — United States. 4. Gynecology — United States. 5. Obstetrics — United States. 6. Gynecology, Operative — United States. 7. Surgery, Unnecessary — United States. I. Title. [DNLM: 1. Internship and residency. 2. Obstetrics — Education. 3. Gynecology — Education. WQ18 S437m]
RG143.A1S37 618'.07'1173 79-27503
ISBN 0-395-29137-2

Printed in the United States of America

S 10 9 8 7 6 5 4 3 2 1

For my mother, Sally Harbinson

Acknowledgments

No one knows fully the experiences and people that have shaped her or his thinking. As a neophyte in medical sociology, I found the insights in Eliot Freidson's *Profession of Medicine* to be particularly significant. I am indebted to Pauline Bart for teaching me critical thinking and for introducing me to the crucial issues in women's health. The research for this book could not have been undertaken or completed without Rue Bucher and, for her years of help and guidance, I am especially grateful. The women's health movement provided the motivation to write this book and continues to be among the more salient influences in my thinking on health care.

It isn't possible to thank everyone who has contributed to this effort but special mention is due those most directly involved. Pauline Bart, Rue Bucher, David Carpenter, James Carey, and Kathleen Crittenden read an early form of the manuscript, and their direction and thoughtful comments were especially important. I also pay thanks to Joyce Basil, Gena Corea, Arlene Kaplan Daniels, Gil Dunn, David Franks, Lenore Gay, Alice Henry, Joe Marolla, Sheryl Burt Ruzek, and Barbara Seaman for their help, advice, and interest.

My friends and colleagues in the Department of Sociology at the University of Illinois at Chicago Circle and in the Department of Sociology and Anthropology at Virginia Commonwealth University supplied support and encouragement that has been very much appreciated.

The excellent typing assistance of Marian Boothe, Mary Kay Gillespie, and Marge Hopkins made the book a physical reality.

Though they are anonymous, I am most grateful for the cooperation extended to me by the residents and other staff members of the Departments of Obstetrics and Gynecology at "Elite Medical Center" and "Mass Hospital." To the women patients at Elite and Mass, a very special thanks.

I am especially indebted to Anita McClellan, of Houghton Mifflin, who edited this book with insight, precision, and patience.

To Sally Harbinson, for her example, I owe more than can be expressed.

The contents of this book do not necessarily reflect the perspective of those mentioned and, naturally, I alone am responsible for the final work.

Contents

Men Who Control Women's Health

Introduction

Men Who Control Women's Health is the result of three fascinating, though difficult, years. During the mid seventies, as a sociologist, I spent hundreds of hours as an observer in labor and delivery rooms, surgical suites, clinics, classes, and informal gatherings at Elite Medical Center and Mass Hospital, the pseudonyms I am using for two hospitals with training programs in obstetrics and gynecology.

In the early seventies, stimulated by the work of several feminists, I had become interested in obstetrician-gynecologists and their control over women's health. To understand "women's doctors," I decided to examine the forces that mold their attitudes and behavior. After a relatively brief period of exposure to the world of residents (as these specialists-in-training are called), it became apparent to me that the most valued experiences were those that occurred in the delivery room or surgical suite. Because of the importance placed by residents on their surgical experience, a large part of my research was devoted to this area. Fortuitously, the startling news about unnecessary operations was soon to break. My study of surgical training revealed attitudes about the efficacy of operative therapy that help to explain the increase in obstetric and gynecologic surgery.

Although surgical training is a major focus of this book, several related issues are also addressed. The profession of obstetrics and gynecology is examined to demonstrate how the practice of medicine and physicians' professional goals interact to influence the development of attitudes and skills that are at variance with the health care needs of women. It is hoped that the demystification of these physicians will arm the consumer with a powerful tool — information. Finally, since this research took place in teaching hospitals, where the poor become "training material" for residents, this book cannot help illustrating the poverty of our health "uncare" institutions. In documenting some of the abuses, I hope to raise questions about the compatability of medical training and patient care under the current system.

This book reflects my background as a sociologist. Consequently, the questions I raise are directed at the social rather than the physiological impact of medicine. My interest in medicine has to do with the social organization of health care, with the role and power relationships between various providers and consumers of services, and with cultural beliefs, attitudes, and values and their effect on health care.

A word of explanation about the research reported in this book is in order. Social scientists typically engage in at least two types of research endeavors. One type is an attempt to verify or test existing theories built on research that has already been done. To accomplish this, the researcher follows certain traditional methodological rules. For example, he or she should investigate a sample of the population that has been randomly selected. If this rule is followed, the researcher is able to claim results that are typical of all similarly defined phenomena.

The second kind of research is an attempt to discover rather than verify theory. Exploratory research, as this type is called, is most applicable to questions about which little is known or to areas in which little theory exists.

An exploratory approach to training in obstetrics and gynecology was chosen for this study because relatively little sociological research has been done on surgeons. Moreover, much of what is available reflects a medical perspective and is biased in favor of physicians.

When the object of an exploratory study is the understanding of behavior, field methods or participant-observation is often used. Because human behavior is assumed to develop through continuous and ever-changing interaction with others, the researcher must get close to the people she or he studies. This can best be accomplished by observing people in their own environment. I therefore spent almost three years with the residents and as nearly as possible tried to experience subjectively the residents' world in an attempt to get an insider's view.

Residents in obstetrics and gynecology were required to spend a certain amount of time in a number of rotations on several services. I spent protracted periods of observation with the residents on each one of the services and observed all the varied activities in which residents engage, including rounds, meetings, classes, interaction with and examination of patients, obstetrical and gynecological surgery, deliveries, and informal peer and staff interaction in various locations, such as clinics, wards, the emergency room, labor and delivery rooms, operating rooms, and lounges. Observation periods were arranged to cover every hour of the day and every day of the week. I kept careful notes while in the field and typed them within twenty-four hours after initial recording. After approximately six months of observation, when I felt I had a basic understanding of each social unit, I interviewed the residents in each program. Some talked for two or three hours, often well into the night.

General results obtained from this type of research are limited because the objects of such a study are seldom chosen randomly or sampled in large numbers and thus may *not* be representative of all similarly defined phenomena. At the same time, though each training program differs from others to some degree, the combination of characteristics represented by Elite Medical Center and Mass Hospital makes their programs sufficiently typical of other training programs across the United States that the results of this study are probably applicable elsewhere. The fact that two somewhat dissimilar training programs produced similar outcomes strengthens the contention made in this book that increasing rates of obstetrical and gynecological surgery are due, in part, to the practice of allowing surgeons-in-training to do unnecessary surgery.

Field research is a rewarding experience, but since the sociologist or anthropologist is almost always cast in the role of an outsider, entering an unfamiliar and sometimes hostile group or culture, she or he inevitably faces problems and hazards not encountered in other types of research endeavors. The two years I had spent working in a hospital while a college undergraduate were a valuable introduction to the world of medicine. Nonetheless, I encountered difficulties in every step of the research, some due to my own mistakes and others to circumstances over which I had no control. For whatever value they may have, I record some of these experiences here.

The first hurdle, which at times made the project appear impossible, was obtaining permission to do the research. Naïvely, I believed at the outset that I would have a choice among a number of institutions with residency programs in obstetrics and gynecology and that the only problem would be to decide which to select among a number of excellent choices. After all, similar studies have been done on training in other medical specialties. In addition, several recent studies that have analyzed social processes in childbirth and maternity necessitated accessibility by researchers to the same facilities that I sought. I was thus surprised to be refused permission to do my research by several institutions that I had believed would be relatively accessible. In retrospect, it is interesting to speculate on the source of the difficulty.

In general, the staffs of both institutions that eventually opened their doors to me were helpful and cooperative. My presence, however, was not welcomed by all. Those who explained their opposition also shed light on the larger issue of social research on the providers, in contrast to the consumers, of health care. That is, although patients are the object of considerable social, psychological, and medical research, some of it drug-related and dangerous, physicians are reluctant to subject themselves even to mild scrutiny. This is understandable; medicine is feeling the pressure of attack from a number of sources. Consumer and patient advocate groups are becoming a vocal force, and the government appears to be moving toward some form of regulatory legislation, thus encroaching on previously closed territory. The profession of obstetrics and gynecology, specifically, has been under criticism by the women's movement, and a study such as this one had the potential of unearthing politically controversial material. As a result of these developments, social researchers can expect greater difficulty gaining admission to the previously somewhat accessible inner circles of the medical establishment.

Ironically, the difficulties I initially encountered ultimately resulted in a better choice of hospitals. The only option, other than giving up, was to try harder for permission at institutions that would have been my first choice had I not believed them to be inaccessible. Persistence was rewarded. After months of delay, permission for me to undertake the research was granted by the Departments of Obstetrics and Gynecology at Elite Medical Center and, somewhat after, at Mass Hospital. The condition was that I guarantee the complete anonymity of the institutions and of all individuals involved. In compliance with that condition, I have substituted descriptive pseudonyms for actual names of the institutions. Because there were so few female residents in each program, I have consistently used the pronoun "he," regardless of actual sex, in order to protect these women's identities.

Once I had been granted permission, I was relatively free to go wherever residents in obstetrics and gynecology would ordinarily be found. But establishing rapport and gaining the cooperation of the residents was another major hurdle. Elite Medical Center posed the greater difficulty primarily because it was the first institution I entered. It was there that the majority of my mistakes were made. By the time I entered Mass, I was a somewhat more sophisticated researcher.

I was introduced to the residents at Elite by a short directive issued by the Department Chair, explaining that a sociologist would be observing them for a period of time in order to do research on surgical training in obstetrics and gynecology. I was introduced to the senior resident on the clinic service, where, it was mutually agreed, I would start my observation. However, it was up to me to break the ice — no easy task in a less than enthusiastic group. The directive had created a difficult atmosphere, particularly because it came from the Chair, who had a reputation among residents for an almost omniscient ability to find out about events and actions he was not present to observe.

> One of the medical students asked me if I was a nurse. I told him that I was a sociologist. He responded, "Oh, you are the person in the famous directive." I asked why it was famous and was told that everyone was talking about it and looking around corners to see if I was following them or investigating them. He asked what the research was about and I told him how doctors learn to be surgeons. He responded that that much was in the directive — what was it really about? (Field Notes, Elite.)

It wasn't until later that I understood the impact of the directive. Clearly, the residents saw me as a spy. On many occasions in the beginning one resident would admonish another to be quiet during a conversation because "she is taking it all down."

For my part, I wasn't doing much to help the situation. Before entering Elite, I had read several accounts of other researchers' experiences in medical settings and expected that mine would parallel theirs. For instance, other researchers suggested it was acceptable to jot down notes in the sight of the participants because hospital staff were accustomed to people, such as medical students, taking notes. However, the first time I attempted to record notes in the presence of residents, the resulting strain was ample discouragement for me not to do it again. The residents reacted whenever they saw me writing in a notebook. Once while I was sitting in a lounge catching up on notes, a resident walked in and quickly remarked that it made him paranoid to see me writing. There was literally only one place in the hospital where I did not run the risk of encountering a resident. It became my practice to repair to the privacy of a stall in a women's washroom when I wanted to record notes.

Why such paranoia? There were several reasons. To begin with, the residents were, in fact, trying to conceal certain information from me. Many times what they were attempting to hide was completely insignificant. Other information, however, was important. Some of the residents had decided that I was "really" studying how they treated institutional patients.

This only partially explains the problem. I believe there is something inherently unnerving or disconcerting about being "watched" while you work and having your words and actions recorded. I had to ask myself how I would feel if the tables were turned. In this sense, though I was unaware of it, other things about me were disturbing to the residents.

I had decided, on entering Elite, that I would be an observer, not a participant. My reasoning was that if I took part in the action, I would somehow change it by my participation and thus would get a distorted view of the residents' world. My style, then, was to remain passively in the background, interjecting as little as possible of myself into a situation. Finally, I realized that my effort to remain aloof was itself distorting the situation. My remaining on the periphery of the group and withholding information about myself created mystery about me. In effect, I was asking the residents to allow me to know them and their social world without giving or revealing anything of myself. Understandably, their reaction was polite resistance. I learned I couldn't observe without participating. I discovered this quite by accident one day in the gynecology clinic:

> A young girl who had never had a pelvic exam and didn't know how to get into the stirrups came into the examining room. Up to this point, I had never touched a patient. But in this case I helped her get into the right position on the table. Dr. S. came in while I was doing this and said, "Good, you are helping us — that must mean that you are sympathetic," and he smiled. I think I have been too remote and too quiet and that was part of the problem.

> This afternoon we had a much friendlier, open conversation and I think I have made some headway with these residents. (Field Notes, Elite.)

After that, I attempted, within limits, to perform small services for the residents. In this way, in their eyes I became part of a collective effort, involved in what they were doing. Having previously worked in a hospital, I was familiar with equipment and routines and could easily run errands, get supplies and equipment, deliver messages, position patients, gown residents in delivery and surgery, and so forth. There is, however, a danger in becoming too involved, because the inclination seems to be to "go native"; that is, to lose objectivity by absorbing the perspective of the group under study. The temptation is probably greater in some situations than others, but it is present to some extent with all groups and is probably a condition necessary to acquiring an insider's knowledge of the behavior studied.

Another important factor is the amount of time spent with the group. Long hours are necessary. I tried to put in as many hours as the residents did and as many days a week. The most hostile resident became friendly when I was still in the delivery room with him at one o'clock on Sunday morning. Residents frequently asked me if I "had to work" that night, forgetting that I wasn't employed by the hospital. They often commented that they hadn't thought anybody worked as many hours as they did.

At various points during my stay, most of the residents accepted me. They stopped cutting off their conversations because I was present and frequently lost track of how long I had been there. For example, residents might ask me if I remembered a case that had occurred two years earlier, long before my time. When I pointed this out, they would respond that it seemed as though I had always been there.

My last task at each institution was to interview the residents, and the long hours I had spent with them were rewarded. They were willing to discuss issues and give information that I believe they would give only to someone who they knew was thoroughly familiar with their world. In discussing unnecessary surgery, for instance, a resident would make a very candid remark and then add, "But you know it happens; you've seen it."

Eventually my role evolved into that of a "social worker." This occurred in response to a dilemma I faced early at Elite. I was frequently present when young and frightened women in the clinics and in labor and delivery reached out for a hand to hold but were met with a stern reprimand from the resident. If I aligned myself with the patients, would I damage my precarious relationship with the residents? That isn't what happened. They interpreted my efforts to quiet and comfort their patients as a gesture of sympathy toward themselves. Obviously, I must understand what a nuisance it was to have to deliver an uncooperative, hysterical teen-ager! It made their job easier, so they were all for it. Despite my efforts to correct the misnomer, they continued to use me as a social worker. For example, late one night a young heroin addict came into the labor and delivery rooms in the final stages of labor. She refused the resident's request for a blood sample, which was needed to test the newborn's addiction. After several unsuccessful attempts at persuasion, the resident called me to talk to the woman.

Ethical considerations were also involved. I saw women talked into surgery they didn't need; I saw procedures forced on women who didn't understand them. Later, I was asked what I did. My honest answer is that I did what I could without upsetting my relationship with the residents. But there is an acceptable limit. Interference beyond a certain point would obviously have resulted in termination of the research. It is my hope that the report of what I found will justify my silence.

• • •

Starting on page 261 is a glossary that the reader can consult for explanations of technical terms.

I

The Problem

American Health Un-Care

In the United States, health care is a dual system; there is one type and quality of services for the middle class and wealthy and another for the medically indigent, who are primarily the nonwhite, poor, and elderly members of society. The duality of the system reflects the class composition of our economic structure and the built-in stratification dividing people into "haves" and "have nots" by an unequal distribution of opportunity, income, and power. Health care is a vivid microcosm of inequality, American style.

To many it seems that health care is a "nonsystem," disorganized, chaotic, and with no one in charge. But as Elliott Krause, author of *Power and Illness*, advised those who think this is the case, "Try to change it."[1]

The tremendous profit of the health care industry explains part of the resistance to change. The corporations that produce drugs, hospital and medical supplies, machines and equipment — the elaborate technology and hardware of medicine — make huge profits, as do physicians, insurance companies, and the nursing home industry.[2] The investment that private industry and the American Medical Association (AMA) have in the status quo would make removing profit from illness a task comparable to the elimination of world conflict.

Health care is also a system in crisis. Although the United States continues to be the only Western industrialized nation without some form of guaranteed national health care, the burden of paying the rising price of medical hardware and hospital and physician fees has become so great that the middle class can't afford to be ill. The medically indigent or "institutional patients" pay in another, perhaps more costly, way. Reduced to using the emergency rooms, inpatient and outpatient clinics, and hospital wards of public and teaching hospitals, where they become the "teaching and experimental material" for physicians-in-training, institutional patients, as this book will illustrate, pay for health care with their bodies.

Health care is a monopoly in the United States controlled by organized medicine and its powerful legislative lobby, the AMA, which has been successful in limiting medical practice to all but a few AMA-sanctioned practitioners.[3] In many states, for example, women are not able to choose between the services of an obstetrician or a nurse-midwife because midwives are barred from the delivery room. But more important, the monopoly over medical knowledge, which is considered too difficult and technical for the average lay person to understand, places the consumer at a decided disadvantage. Even the average, well-informed individual is handicapped in evaluating a physician's advice or performance because the information needed to make an informed decision is withheld or unavailable.

Who's in Control?

Because the health care consumer, especially when ill, is vulnerable and potentially open to exploitation, physicians are morally mandated to act according to a code of ethics. But, increasingly, reports of such practices as "ghost surgery," in which, without the patient's knowledge or consent, residents (surgeons-in-training) are substituted for surgeons, and the frequent reports of unnecessary surgery raise a question about the adequacy of ethics alone as a protection for consumers. That many believe patient advocates are necessary seems to indicate that from the consumer's perspective there is a serious flaw in the system.

A potentially more important question concerns the monitoring of physician performance. Of all professions, medicine has been among the most successful in achieving autonomy and establishing the freedom to work without regulation from outside its own community. Consumers have a very small voice in policies that regulate the terms of health care delivery, and only physicians control the content of medical work and the education of recruits. This autonomy means that it is only physicians who are in a position to monitor each other's behavior and performance.

The traditional "solo fee-for-service" pattern of medical practice, with individual entrepreneurs isolated in one-"man" practices, reduced the observability of medical work, a condition obviously necessary for monitoring. Group practice, becoming more common today, permits more visibility. But the fact remains that, unlike other professions, such as teaching, medicine is primarily practiced in private. In either the solo or group type of practice, sociologist Eliot Freidson[4] argues, the most severe form of punishment is "referral boycott," refusing to refer patients to an erring physician. A boycott, however, does not prevent a physician from practicing medicine if patients can be obtained from some other source. Furthermore, Freidson points out, such a boycott results in less, not more, observability, because the physician becomes even more isolated. The extent to which physicians use this method of colleague regulation is questionable anyway. Since referral relationships tend to be reciprocal, a boycott could mean the termination of a lucrative source of patients for the boycotting physician. Evidence also suggests that physicians are reluctant to exercise control over a colleague's performance. Even in large medical organizations, where observability is at its greatest, the most severe form of regulation seems to be "talking to" or "giving advice," which, of course, can be ignored.[5]

Perhaps the most disturbing evidence of the lack of regulation among physicians is reported by Marcia Millman in her book

The Unkindest Cut: Life in the Backrooms of Medicine.[6] In order to understand the way in which physicians handle medical mistakes, Millman studied Mortality Review Conferences. These conferences are held by a board of hospital physicians who meet periodically to discuss medical cases that ended in an in-hospital patient death and in which there is some question of error, failure, or mismanagement on the part of the physicians involved. Millman's research took place in teaching hospitals, where there is more regulation than in nonteaching hospitals, and involved a "better than average" group of physicians.

Although the purpose of a review is to detect mistakes and prevent their reoccurrence, the researcher found that the reviews often served to justify an error and remove physician responsibility for it, usually by blaming the victim for not following orders. Millman discovered that during the meetings, physician after physician would testify how he was led to the same mistaken judgment, thereby providing justification and spreading responsibility so that no individual doctor was made to look guilty. Moreover, some controversial cases were not reviewed at all. The chief of medicine at one hospital reported that 80 percent of the errors were simply ignored, that he could choose only "certain" cases to present, and that the conferences had turned into a cordial affair among colleagues. Millman argues that in the matter of peer regulation, physicians follow the golden rule: knowing they have made similar errors and are likely to make more, they are reluctant to criticize a colleague.

An expression of consumer alarm is warranted because, as Freidson observed, "the medical profession, which gained freedom from regulation by others, regulates itself in ways whose effectiveness is not self-evident."[7]

If physicians do not regulate each other, we must assume they are self-regulating. Consequently, an important source of control on physician behavior is the socialization that occurs during medical training. During the years spent in medical school, internship, and residency, physicians-in-training acquire not only the technical and cognitive skills of their profession, but also the values and ethics that will guide their behavior once they are out of the protected training environment.

Men Who Control Women's Health is about surgical training at Elite Medical Center and Mass Hospital. Readers may be surprised by what takes place in the corridors and back rooms of teaching hospitals, as well as by the attitudes of the people who train there. This glimpse behind the scenes provides insight into physician behavior in private practice and helps to explain unnecessary surgery, an issue of particular significance to women.

Are Women the Sicker Sex?

Issues related to health care and physician performance are particularly significant to women because women consume a large proportion of medical services. In 1974, not counting visits accompanying patient-children, women's office visits to physicians were 44 percent higher than men's.[8] Although the average life expectancy is longer for women than for men, according to surveys conducted by the government, females report more acute and chronic illnesses even when disorders due to pregnancy and childbirth are not counted.[9] Gove and Tudor,[10] working from community surveys of mental illness and data on outpatient care and admissions to psychiatric facilities, concluded, in addition, that all of the pertinent information suggests more women than men seek psychiatric treatment.

The seemingly contradictory picture of women's health — more illness but a longer life expectancy — has been the object of some speculation. Essentially, three types of explanations, each related to women's social roles, have been offered.[11] Some suggest that the difference in female and male illness rates reflect the greater social acceptance of weakness and help-seeking behavior for women. The traditional male role, in contrast, demands toughness and discourages the kind of dependency that the sick role encourages. Others state that women display more illness and sick-role behavior because it is more consistent with other female-role obligations but is not compatible with those of men. They argue (perhaps unrealistically) that it is easier for a woman who works in the home to assume the sick role than it is for the traditional male breadwinner, who works outside the home, to do so. Still others argue that women are, in fact, the sicker sex, not because their social roles allow for illness behavior, but because the stresses associated with the female role create illness.

Debate aside, for our purposes, the important point is that women are frequently in touch with physicians and the health care system. Especially during her reproductive years, the woman consults obstetrician-gynecologists for routine prenatal, postnatal, and gynecological care, birth control information, and abortion service. Of all types of physicians, then, the obstetrician-gynecologists, specialists whom women consult even when they are in good health, have been among the most intimately involved in female health care. This observation is reflected in a recent statement by the American College of Obstetricians and Gynecologists (ACOG) in which it claimed that it was "the spokesman for women's health care." This, in turn, prompted a quick reply from feminists, who argue that surgical specialists are not prepared to meet the overall health needs of women.

Those women who prefer a female obstetrician-gynecologist, or any type of female physician, will hardly be surprised to learn such a doctor has been a rarity in the United States. Occupational segregation in health care, like the larger occupational structure, traditionally crowds females into lower-paying occupations, and prestigious professions remain largely the domain of white males. So, for example, in 1970, 93.1 percent of physicians were male, and 97.3 percent of registered nurses were female.[12] The percentage of women in obstetrics and gynecology is even less than in medicine generally. In 1974, among the 15,927 members of the ACOG, only 568, or 3.5 percent, were women.[13] With 96.5 percent of the profession male, the majority of American women currently do not have the choice of female obstetrician-gynecologists.

Since obstetrics and gynecology would seem to be a natural choice for women entering medicine, the fact that female medical students choose to specialize in other areas of medicine makes an interesting and a strong statement about the specialty.

Traditionally, the long hours required of a busy obstetrician, which made the field seem incompatible with childbearing and child-rearing, were thought to be a deterrent to women — and to some men. This disadvantage, however, is rapidly diminishing because of the current shift to group practice.

A recent study[14] of female medical students at the University of Vermont Medical School makes it clear that other factors than long hours are deterrents. The women medical students in Vermont were concerned about the way the specialty relates to women; they either wished to enter the profession to change it or were "so upset by the way gynecologists are seen to interreact with women that they want little to do with the specialty."[15]

Women are underrepresented in all of the surgical specialties, not just obstetrics and gynecology. However, as the Vermont study asserts, it is not the surgery per se that bothers women, but the antifeminist attitudes they have encountered in the operating rooms. The authors conclude, "Until women medical students perceive Obstetrics and Gynecology as a profession which is genuinely interested in women's problems, they will continue to be more attracted to Family Practice, Pediatrics and Psychiatry where their particular humanistic qualities are welcomed."[16]

The residents at Elite and Mass referred to obstetrics and gynecology as "the happy specialty" because most of the problems encountered are curable, and women, because they are cured, are presumed to be happy and grateful. But there is evidence to suggest that this is far too optimistic a view. The frequency of articles about women's health, in magazines from *Ms.* to *Woman's Day*, and best-selling books like *Our Bodies, Ourselves*, by the Boston Women's Health Book Collective, indicate that women of all backgrounds are interested in and concerned about their health care. The women's health movement, with its self-help ideology, is another indication that some women are critical of the care they receive.

Unfortunately, there is good reason for the interest and concern. Latest government statistics show that the hysterectomy has become the number one operation in the United States and now outranks the tonsillectomy and the appendectomy, the former top surgical contenders. Recent AMA-sponsored research placed the hysterectomy and dilation and curettage (D & C) second among unnecessary procedures, surpassed only by surgery on the knee.[17] Since gynecologists seemingly regard the uterus as an expendable organ, useless for purposes other than childbearing, they have a casual attitude about its removal. Some even go so far as to recommend prophylactic hysterectomies, surgery in the complete absence of any disease at all. Equally disturbing, according to a 1977 editorial in the *New England Journal of Medicine,* some physicians are recommending prophylactic mastectomies[18] for women with "precancerous" breast disease, despite the admission that "there is disagreement about what constitutes 'premalignant' changes in the breast."[19]

Sexism in Medicine

During the past several years, increasing attention has been paid to the issue of sexism in medicine as accumulating evidence indicates that biases in the male-dominated profession do affect medical treatment and patient care.

In 1972, with the publication of her popular *Free and Female,*[20] Barbara Seaman raised a number of important issues. Why, Seaman asked, "are American women shaved, humiliated, drugged, painted and stuck up into stirrups to deliver their babies?" Why are women given birth control pills and IUDs without being informed of the dangers? How many hysterectomies are of the "hip pocket variety," where the main benefit accrues to the surgeon's wallet? Providing some answers, Seaman hoped, would help liberate women from their gynecologists.

Again in 1977, Seaman, this time writing with her physician-husband, Gideon Seaman, published a landmark book that should be required reading for every woman. *Women and the Crisis in Sex Hormones*[21] is an ambitious documentation of the potentially dangerous effects of the estrogens that millions of women ingest daily in the form of birth control pills and estrogen replacement therapy (ERT).[22] The history of diethylstilbestrol (DES), sometimes called stilbestrol, a synthetic estrogen, is one disturbing example among several presented by the Seamans that show the disregard with which these dangerous estrogens have been forced on a trusting female population.

From the early 1940s until 1971, DES was prescribed by obstetricians for pregnant women who were suspected of being prone to miscarriage. Some women, who took the drug experimentally, weren't told the truth about what they were taking. They were told the drug was a vitamin. As a result, information that might have prevented them from participating in the experiments was withheld.

By 1967, it had been established that DES was a carcinogen in animals, but it wasn't until November 1971 that the Food and Drug Administration (FDA) finally took steps to restrict its use in pregnant women. An illustration of the time-bomb effect of estrogen is that, years later, some daughters of DES mothers are suffering cancer of the vagina and cervix at a rate in excess of the rest of the female population in their age range. There is no reliable way to predict how many will develop cancer later in life. Problems have also been detected in some sons of DES mothers. There appears to be a higher rate than normal of sterility, caused in several cases by a malformation of the spermatic duct system.

Unfortunately, the story didn't end in 1971. As the Seamans report, DES, now indisputedly known to be a human carcinogen, is still prescribed for women. Although it took until 1977, the *Physician's Desk Reference* does now carry the following warning in large caps: THIS DRUG PRODUCT (DES) SHOULD NOT BE

USED AS A POSTCOITAL CONTRACEPTIVE. But despite the warning and the dangers, DES in the form of "the morning-after pill" is still in use. The irony of the tragedy is that it has never really been established that DES prevents miscarriage (when taken in small doses over extended periods of time) or prevents conception (when taken in large doses over a brief period of time). So some of the women who are given the morning-after pill will conceive and will expose their fetuses to DES, as will some of the rape victims who are given the pill in hospital emergency rooms without being tested to see if they are already pregnant.

In the same year that Seaman published *Free and Female,*[23] Ellen Frankfort coined the term "vaginal politics." Her book of the same title described the frustration of coping with a health care system that treats women like children and denies them the opportunity to acquire the information necessary to make informed decisions. Advocating the simple yet revolutionary idea of female-centered self-help, Frankfort urged women to arm themselves with a speculum, learn about their bodies, participate in self-help groups, and take control of their reproductive lives.

Since the publication of these classics, other voices have been raised against sexism in medicine. Psychiatry, with its emphasis on traditional roles for women and sexist notions of what constitutes a healthy female psyche, has been criticized,[24] and dissatisfaction with obstetrics and gynecology has been strong enough to launch the women's health movement. A few dissenting voices have even come from within the profession. Writing in the *American Journal of Obstetrics and Gynecology,* Barbara Kaiser and her husband, Irwin Kaiser, a gynecologist, point out that gynecologists have always treated women as though they were children. The challenge the women's movement offers to gynecology, the Kaisers argue, is "the demand that female patients be treated like full human beings, and that no female patient of any age be required, tacitly or overtly, to conform to demeaning and insulting role stereotypes . . . It is also time for gynecologists to give up the assumption of innate superiority and of omniscience that they have so long enjoyed."[25]

An ambitious documentation of sexism in medicine is Gena Corea's recent *The Hidden Malpractice.*[26] In it, Corea describes how men came to dominate medicine, and demonstrates the effect of that domination on the types of theories constructed to explain women's problems.

In a parody on male-constructed theories, Corea asks whether men would be considered unreasonable for questioning theories that women might construct about them if medicine were female-dominated. What if female physicians decided that "the monthly change in man's testosterone level so upsets his emotional equilibrium that he is unqualified for professional jobs" or that "failure to accept the male role causes many of men's abdominal pains." Yet similar statements are frequent in the gynecology literature. For example, "Premenstrual tension produces an oppressive, cyclic cloud which prevents women from functioning in a smooth, logical male fashion."[27]

• • •

In a classic essay, Irving Kenneth Zola[28] argued that medicine has become an institution of social control. As more of daily life becomes medicalized, supposedly morally neutral and objective physicians are able to make, in the name of health and illness, final judgments that pertain to an ever-increasing part of human existence. Their unquestioned status as experts has resulted in their almost unprecedented power over people's lives.

Obstetrician-gynecologists are an excellent case in point. Designated the official and legitimate experts on the female reproductive tract, they have also been successful in broadening their sphere of influence to include the female sex role, psychology, and sexuality, despite the fact that these are areas in which they have no particular expertise and which they tend to interpret from a decidedly male point of view. A reading of gynecology textbooks is instructive on this point. For example, a 1971 text by a Harvard gynecologist carried the following advice:

> If the sexual inadequacy on the part of the wife stems from a fundamental immaturity and inability or failure to assume the normal adult female role in the marital relationship, he [the gynecologist] may be able to help by gradually imparting to her the nature of what her role should be — as Sturgis has described it so well, the fact that although the instinctive sexual drive of the male, who carries the primary responsibility for biologic survival of the race, is greater than hers, it is nevertheless of fundamental importance for the woman, his wife, particularly in a monogamous society, to make herself available for the fulfillment of this drive, and perfectly natural and normal that she do it willingly and derive satisfaction and pleasure from the union. Herein lies her power and purpose — to preserve the family unit as a happy, secure place for both man and wife and for the rearing of their children. Only by understanding and assuming this role can a woman throw off childhood inhibitions and taboos and attain the feminine maturity essential to a happy, successful marital adjustment.[29]

What action is available to the woman concerned about her health care? Corea urges women to overcome their traditional sex-role learning, which encourages passivity and dependence on men, and to begin taking responsibility for their own health care. Admittedly, this is a difficult task when information is either unavailable or shrouded by medical mystery. Informed consumers have a definite advantage in the marketplace. Let us hope this book about the profession of obstetrics and gynecology, its history and contemporary practices, will remove a little more of the mystery.

Notes

1. Elliott Krause, *Power and Illness: The Political Sociology of Health and Medical Care* (New York: Elsevier, 1977), p. 154.

2. See for example, David Kotelchuck, ed., *Prognosis Negative* (New York: Vintage Books, 1976), and Barbara Ehrenreich and John Ehrenreich, *The American Health Empire: Power, Profits and Politics* (New York: Vintage Books, 1971).
3. For an analysis of the medical profession, see Eliot Freidson, *Profession of Medicine* (New York: Dodd, Mead and Company, 1973).
4. Eliot Freidson, *Professional Dominance: The Social Structure of Medical Care* (New York: Atherton Press, 1970).
5. See Eliot Freidson and Buford Rhea, "Processes of Control in a Company of Equals," *Social Problems,* 11 (1963), 119–131, and Mary E. H. Goss, "Influence and Authority among Physicians in an Outpatient Clinic," *American Sociological Review,* 26 (1961), 39–50.
6. Marcia Millman, *The Unkindest Cut: Life in the Backrooms of Medicine* (New York: William Morrow & Co., 1977).
7. Freidson, *Professional Dominance,* p. 95.
8. United States Department of Health, Education, and Welfare, Health United States, No. (HRA) 77–1232, 1977, p. 257.
9. Lois M. Verbrugge, "Females and Illness: Recent Trends in Sex Differences in the United States," *Journal of Health and Social Behavior,* 17 (1976), 387–403.
10. Walter Gove and Jeannette Tudor, "Adult Sex Roles and Mental Illness," *American Journal of Sociology,* 78 (1973), 812–835.
11. Constance Nathanson, "Illness and the Feminine Role: A Theoretical Review," *Social Science and Medicine,* 9 (1975), 57–62.
12. Vicente Navarro, "Women in Health Care," *New England Journal of Medicine,* 292 (1975), 398-402.
13. Barbara L. Kaiser and Irwin H. Kaiser, "The Challenge of the Women's Movement to American Gynecology," *American Journal of Obstetrics and Gynecology,* 120 (1974), 652–665.
14. Mary Jane Gray and Jayne Ackerman, "Attitudes of Women Medical Students Toward Obstetrics and Gynecology," *Journal of the American Medical Women's Association,* 33 (1978), 162–164.
15. Ibid., p. 163.
16. Ibid.
17. For a more detailed account of unnecessary hysterectomies, see Chapter IV.
18. This is a procedure in which breast tissue is removed but the nipple and areola are preserved so that the breast can be artificially reconstructed by, for example, the use of silicone implants.
19. I am indebted to Gena Corea for calling this to my attention. Robert M. Goldwyn, "Subcutaneous Mastectomy," *New England Journal of Medicine,* 297 (1977), 503.
20. Barbara Seaman, *Free and Female* (New York: Coward, McCann & Geoghegan, 1972).

21. Barbara Seaman and Gideon Seaman, *Women and the Crisis in Sex Hormones* (New York: Rawson Associates, 1977).
22. See Chapter IV for more information on ERT.
23. Ellen Frankfort, *Vaginal Politics* (New York: Quadrangle Books, 1972).
24. See, for example, Pauline Bart and Diana Scully, "The Politics of Hysteria," in *Gender and Disordered Behavior,* Edith Gomberg and Violet Franks, eds. (Larchmont, New York: Bruner/Mazel, 1979); Inge K. Broverman, et al., "Sex Role Stereotypes and Clinical Judgments of Mental Health," *Journal of Consulting and Clinical Psychology,* 34 (1970), 1–7; Phyllis Chesler, *Women and Madness* (New York: Doubleday, 1972); Joseph Marolla and Diana Scully, "Rape and Psychiatric Vocabularies of Motive," in *Gender and Disordered Behavior.*
25. Kaiser and Kaiser, "The Challenge of the Women's Movement," 659–660.
26. Gena Corea, *The Hidden Malpractice: How American Medicine Treats Women as Patients and Professionals* (New York: William Morrow, 1977).
27. Robert A. Kinch, "Response to Kaiser and Kaiser," *American Journal of Obstetrics and Gynecology,* 120 (1974), 664.
28. Irving Kenneth Zola, "Medicine as an Institution of Social Control," in *The Cultural Crisis of Modern Medicine,* John Ehrenreich, ed. (New York: Monthly Review Press, 1978).
29. Thomas H. Green, *Gynecology: Essentials of Clinical Practice* (Boston: Little, Brown, 1971), p. 436.

II

"Baby Catchers and Uterus Snatchers"

"BABY CATCHER AND UTERUS SNATCHER" is medical slang for obstetrician-gynecologist; it reflects the belief that, compared with other areas of medicine, the work is boring and routine. Such was not always the case. In the early days, before their common interest in the female pelvis joined them into one specialty, obstetricians and gynecologists had the reputation of being surgical innovators. What follows is an attempt to place male-dominated medicine within the context of eighteenth- and nineteenth-century American values and to examine the significant trends and controversies in preanesthesia midwifery and pelvic surgery. During this period the pattern was set for twentieth-century obstetric and gynecologic practices, and the role of the modern woman's doctor was defined.

Cultural Customs and Childbirth

Medical customs differ from society to society because they are affected by the cultural context in which they develop. Niles Newton[1] notes that all known cultures have customs concerning appropriate behavior during pregnancy and labor. These customs are dependent, to some degree, on the culturally patterned beliefs of the birth attendants. Cultural patterning determines attitudes about childbearing and also regulates the major aspects of reproduction, including diet during pregnancy, type of help given childbearing women, birth position, and the spacing of children.[2] Childbirth, then, provides an interesting example of the impact of culture on a physiological process. To understand what happened to American childbirth, it is necessary to trace the history of American obstetrics.

Nineteenth-Century Men-Midwives

For most of recorded history and in many parts of the world today, women-midwives[3] assist in the act of giving birth. It has been only in recent times and primarily in the United States that childbirth has been attended exclusively by physicians, most of whom are men. Largely because men-midwives — as the early obstetricians were called — wanted to establish obstetrics as a proper and necessary medical specialty, childbirth was redefined. Instead of being a natural event, it became a medical problem requiring surgical expertise. Facilitated by the refinement of the cesarean section and by the invention of the obstetrical forceps — a surgical technique and a surgical tool of which physicians claimed exclusive knowledge — medicine waged a bitter battle against the popular "granny" midwife, and in the process imposed new, medically oriented customs on childbirth.

Nineteenth-century efforts by American medicine to control childbirth were chiefly those of general practitioners, with little specific training, who conducted home deliveries. Early in that century, the encroachment of medicine into midwifery met with some resistance from among its own male ranks. Objections took two forms. The first can be traced to the remnants of Victorian morality, which made physical contact with the female genitalia an odious task for physicians and an indiscretion on the part of women who permitted it. Although motherhood was the socially accepted role for women, it was obvious that women who filled that role had had sexual intercourse. Pregnancy was a symbol of the sexual nature that "good" women were supposed to suppress or conceal, and it caused embarrassment to themselves as well as to physicians.

Writing around 1848, Dr. Samuel Gregory noted that the first use of a male-midwife was in 1663 by the Duchess of Villiers, "a favorite mistress of Louis XIV of France." Modern women, in Gregory's opinion, were following a precedent set 185 years before by a court prostitute and were inviting a "violent attack against chastity." But even the duchess had "some modest scruples"; she wore a hood over her head whenever a male attended her.[4] There were other types of modesty-preserving devices that protected the delicate sensibility of man-midwife and patient.[5] A delivery position was used in which the woman was placed on her side so that the man-midwife, working from behind, could avoid eye contact. Some men-midwives covered themselves and patient with a sheet, their work apparently not hindered by the dark, and one man-midwife is reported to have disguised himself as a woman by wearing a ruffled nightcap and gown.[6]

Petitioning physicians to "give it [midwifery] up, whatever might be the pecuniary sacrifice," Samuel Gregory, as well as other physicians, believed that

> the introduction of men into the lying-in chamber, in place of female attendants, has increased the suffering and dangers of childbearing women, and brought multiplied injuries and fatalities upon mothers and children; it violates the sensitive feelings of husbands and wives, and causes an untold amount of domestic misery; the unlimited intimacy between a numerous profession and the female population silently and effectually wears away female delicacy and professional morality, and tends, probably more than any other cause in existence, to undermine the foundation of public virtue.[7]

A second obstacle facing acceptance of men-midwives was the belief that medical intervention in childbirth was unnecessary and often harmful. Many physicians felt that unless the fetus was in an unnatural position, women-midwives were competent to assist in childbirth, and even ridiculed the idea of employing physicians. A professor at the University of Edinburgh compared men-midwives to a species of frog in which the male draws the ova from the female. If this is a fact, he proclaimed, "this frog practice is doubtless the only precedent, in the whole animal kingdom, in favor of accoucheurs and male-midwifery."[8]

In normal childbirth, granny midwives were at least as skilled and certainly more experienced than physicians. But in the small percentage of complicated deliveries, childbirth could be a frightening and painful experience for women, regardless of who was in attendance. If the fetus lay in an abnormal position, obstructing birth, or if the pelvis was too narrow to permit passage of the fetus, childbirth meant excruciating labor pain and often death for women and fetus. Prior to about 1860, the time that anesthesia came into general use, there was little relief for normal birth pain. The cesarean section was no solution for birth complications, since the operation was fatal for the woman and was therefore used for centuries as a method of delivering a child after the death of the mother.[9]

Men-midwives invented and experimented with an array of instruments to accomplish difficult deliveries. Craniotomies were performed with an instrument called a perforator, which was used to perforate the fetal skull and excavate the contents, thus reducing the size of the head and allowing the fetus's passage through the pelvis. There were also hooks and breaking-and-cutting instruments used to perform an embryotomy, in which the fetus was dissected and extracted in pieces.[10]

Obstetrical forceps, when their use was indicated and they were properly handled, had the potential for averting some of the deaths in childbirth. The instrument was invented around 1695 by the Chamberlen family, who kept its design secret from the medical community in order to increase the personal profits of the family. It was not until 1813 that the "Chamberlen Secret" was finally revealed, moving one practitioner to comment, "He who keeps secret so beneficial an instrument as the harmless obstetrical forceps deserves to have a worm devour his vitals for all eternity."[11]

Women-midwives, perceiving the danger to both their clients and their profession, fought against instrument-aided childbirth or, as it was sometimes called, "meddlesome midwifery." English-born Elizabeth Nihell, a famous eighteenth-century midwife, led such an attack. In a paper titled *A Treatise on the Art of Midwifery, Setting Forth various Abuses therein, especially as to the Practice with Instruments, the whole serving to put all Rational Inquirers in a fair way of very safely forming their Own Judgement upon the Question which is it best to employ in Cases of Pregnancy and Lying-In, a Man-Midwife or a Midwife,* she wrote,

> My very natural and strong attachment to the profession which I have long exercised, created in me an insuppressible indignation at the errors and pernicious innovations introduced into it, and every day gaining ground, under the protection of Fashion, sillily fostering a preference of men to women in the practice of midwifery.[12]

In order for obstetrics to establish its claim and eliminate women-midwives, childbirth, whether complicated or normal, had to be considered a pathological state requiring the intervention of obstetricians and their instruments and surgical techniques. Prospective mothers, as well as the medical community, which tended to view the obstetrician's work as unimportant, had to be convinced that normal pregnancy and childbirth were exceptions and that to consider them normal physiological events was fallacious. Not only was it necessary to establish the validity of surgical techniques in childbirth; it was essential to present the techniques as being safe only in the hands of a surgeon. American medicine claimed it possessed special expertise and the ability to improve prenatal care and to reduce maternal and neonatal mortality. The task that confronted the new profession was proving these claims. Since medicine generally and obstetrics specifically were still at a relatively primitive level of development, their ability to deliver improved care was debatable.

One factor that made men-midwives' claim of improved care dubious was the crude skill they possessed with the newly developed obstetrical instruments. Forceps, especially as used in the nineteenth century, were not harmless. In their book on the history of childbirth in America, Richard Wertz and Dorothy Wertz point out that current obstetrical technique favors the application of "low" forceps in which the fetus's head is low in the birth canal and already visible. Two hundred years ago, men-midwives used "high" forceps, applied before the fetal head was engaged in the mother's pelvis, and "mid" forceps, in which the head was engaged but not yet visible. "These latter operations presented extreme danger to both mother and child, the possibilities of physical damage, infection in damaged tissue, hemorrhage, and a crushed fetal head."[13]

In addition, according to eighteenth- and nineteenth-century reports, unnecessary and experimental use of the instruments, which resulted in injuries, was not uncommon. Dr. Gregory wrote:

> The reader is aware by this time that various instruments are made use of in obstetric practice . . . These instruments are all very useful when it is proper to use them; it is of course proper to use them when it is necessary . . . There is a great propensity in many accoucheurs [men-midwives] to try their dexterity in the use of these mechanical "improvements." In their admiration of instruments and their spirit for action, they follow in the footsteps of their immortal predecessor, Dr. Slop.[14]

It was Gregory's belief that men-midwives were sometimes guilty of malpractice, performing the more complicated craniotomy and embryotomy on the poor for experimental purposes and on the middle class and wealthy because a higher fee could be charged. He stated, "What is most unaccountable . . . is, that when they have wounded the mother, killed the infant, and with violent torture and inexpressible pain, extracted it by piecemeal, they think no reward sufficient for such an extraordinary piece of mangled work."[15]

Although the procedures sometimes were done to save the mother's life, critics, including some physicians, argued that much of the operative interference was a tactic used to establish obstetrics as a necessary surgical specialty. The more surgery and instruments were used, the more it appeared they were necessary. In *The Married Woman's Private Medical Companion,* published in 1847, Dr. A. M. Mauriceau alerted his readers.

> I have long labored under the conviction, that the office of attending women in their confinement should be entrusted to prudent females. There is not, according to my experience, and the reports of the most eminent surgeons, more than one case in three thousand that requires the least assistance. I am aware, however, that there are crafty physicians who attempt, and often succeed, in causing the distressed and alarmed female to believe that it would be altogether impossible for her to get over her troubles without their assistance; and, for the purpose of making it appear that their services are absolutely necessary, they will be continually interfering, sometimes with their instruments, when there is not the least occasion for it. There is no doubt in my mind but that one half of the women attended by these men are delivered before their proper period; and this is the reason why we see so many deformed children, and meet with so many females who have incurable complaints.[17]

As a result of the sometimes inept and needless use of these instruments, women often suffered not only extremely painful childbirth but damage to internal organs as well. Among the worst of these injuries was the vesicovaginal fistula, which can be caused by obstetrical instruments or by prolonged labor. This injury, which is a tear in the wall between the vagina and bladder, resulting in a continuous seepage of urine, caused severe discomfort, unpleasant odors, and often ended in social isolation for the victim.

Added to the problems caused by instruments was the epidemic of puerperal fever, or childbed fever, throughout the

United States and Europe during the nineteenth century. Convincing evidence supplied by an American physician, Oliver Wendell Holmes, before 1840 supported the idea that puerperal fever was contagious, transmitted by hands, clothes, or instruments from an infected woman to a healthy one. The increasing practice of confining women to lying-in hospitals, they contended, heightened the probability of spreading infection. In fact, physicians resisted Holmes's ideas, even ridiculed him, and accepted high mortality rates in lying-in hospitals as normal.

It was a Hungarian physician, Ignaz Semmelweis, who discovered the cause of childbed fever and, in doing so, incurred the wrath of medical colleagues who resented the suggestion that physicians were the conveyers of disease. He observed, as others had before him, that the mortality rate of women in his hospital was three times greater in the clinic that trained medical students than in the clinic that trained midwives. Women were also aware of this and pleaded to be treated by midwives. "Women who were directed to the first clinic [in which medical students worked] wept bitterly, prayed to be allowed to die at home, and gave themselves up for lost."[18] Reasoning that the only difference between the two clinics was that medical students worked in dissection rooms on cadavers as well as on the wards, Semmelweis instructed the students to scrub their hands before touching patients. The death rate fell in his wards from 11.4 percent in 1846 to 1.27 percent in 1848. He concluded that childbed fever was conveyed through the agency of examining fingers. It wasn't, however, until around 1885 that techniques for assuring antiseptic conditions came into general use in American hospitals. Until that time, the mortality rate from puerperal fever was very high in lying-in facilities, often reaching epidemic proportions.

The controversy surrounding women-midwives raged on during the opening decades of the twentieth century. In 1910 in the United States approximately 50 percent of all births were still reported by women-midwives. At the same time, the maternal death rate was the third highest of all countries that kept such records.[19] Medical journals of the period carried numerous articles on the "midwife problem." In them, obstetricians charged that women-midwives were "hopelessly dirty, ignorant, and incompetent,"[20] and were responsible for the high rates of maternal death from puerperal sepsis.[21] Unlike contemporary nurse-midwives, the granny midwife was medically untrained, though greatly experienced in childbirth. In spite of the obstetricians' claim that maternal death rates were reduced, research during that period revealed that the medical profession still lost as many women in childbirth as did women-midwives.[22] A 1912 study of obstetrics education in 120 medical schools revealed the urgent need for reform. The study concluded that medical schools were inadequately equipped and professors poorly prepared for teaching obstetrics. As a result, their students were not prepared to practice obstetrics on graduation. Moreover, one half of the schools reported that ordinary practitioners lost proportionately as many women from puerperal infection as did midwives, and over three-quarters stated that more deaths occurred each year from operations improperly performed by practitioners than from infection in the hands of midwives. The report concluded, "Reform is urgently needed and can be accomplished more speedily by radical improvement in medical education than by attempting the almost impossible task of improving midwives."[23]

Interestingly, obstetricians, who were themselves incompetent, saw the elimination of women-midwives and the expansion of obstetrics as the solution to high infant-mortality rates. A small faction believed the problem would be better handled by training and licensing women midwives. One spokesperson for the American Association for the Study and Prevention of Infant Mortality argued, "If the [woman-] midwife does better work untrained than the general practitioner, what type of work would she do after six months or one year of careful training?"[24] For the most part, the medical profession argued that women-midwives should not be allowed to practice. As another spokesperson put it:

> Some 30,000 women have taken enough practice away from the physician to obtain a livelihood. Unquestionably

> the field of the physician has been invaded and the community is the loser because this form of practitioner is a make-shift, admittedly incapable of coping with the abnormalities of pregnancy, labor, and the puerperium. The more midwives there are and the more successful they are, just so much the worse for the community at large which is thereby being supplied by second-class service.[25]

Though obstetricians argued that their business was reduced by women-midwives, it is doubtful that the profession was adequate to handle the women-midwives' share of childbirth. Women-midwives attended primarily poor and immigrant women, many of whom were accustomed to female birth attendants in their home country and had biases against hospitals and male-conducted childbirth. Social historian G. J. Barker-Benfield points out that the exclusion of women-midwives also meant that a large volume of obstetrical practice would have to go to general practitioners, who by definition had less specialized experience than midwives or obstetricians and who also were the product of shockingly inferior medical education, as revealed by the famous 1910 Flexner report on medical education in the United States and Canada.[26] However, as the emerging profession of obstetrics saw it, not only was the volume of business decreased by women-midwives but, since their clients were mostly poor and working-class women, the "material" with which to train new generations of obstetricians was also diminished.

> The 50 percent of all cases handled by midwives were useless for advancing obstetrical knowledge. Elevating the midwife and training her would decrease the number of cases in which the stethoscope, pelvimeter, and other newly developed or newly applied techniques could be used to increase obstetrical knowledge.[27]

Part of the solution to the "midwife problem" was the establishment of large hospital–medical school complexes with obstetrics clinics and lying-in facilities. Early-nineteenth-century hospitals were often overcrowded and dirty and intended largely for the poor and homeless. Although humanitarian concerns motivated some physicians, it was also true that hospitals for the poor provided a constant supply of clients who could be used for clinical observation, experimentation, and instruction. Then as now, people unable to afford private physician fees received care that was free or at reduced cost in return for providing medicine with "training material." Thus, with one stroke two objectives could be achieved. The need for women-midwives among the poor would be eliminated, and students would be provided with ample "material" on which to train.[28]

Ultimately, women-midwives couldn't compete with the growing power of organized medicine. Although in rural poverty areas, especially in the South, where physicians have always been scarce, granny midwives and home deliveries were never completely eliminated,[29] through campaigns designed to emphasize the dangers of pregnancy and delivery and through restrictive legislation midwives were forced to yield their role in childbirth to physicians.[30] By 1930 home deliveries had declined dramatically, as women, convinced that birth was safer and less painful in hospitals, switched from women-midwives to obstetricians.

Modern Obstetrical Intervention

With the nearly complete elimination of women-midwives, childbirth entered the machine age and the sterile, technologically oriented environment of American hospitals. Presaged by the Chamberlen forceps, birth came under the domination of new experts who not only perceived the process as problematic rather than natural but who were also surgeons trained to intervene.

The International Childbirth Education Association entitled its 1972 special report *The Cultural Warping of Childbirth*[31] in order to draw attention to various obstetrical practices rooted in hospital and medical tradition rather than in scientific research or human physiology. The author, Doris Haire, an officer of the association, presents chilling statistics indicating that Sweden and the Netherlands have the lowest incidence of infant deaths per 1000 live births, but the United States continues to rank fifteenth among the developed countries in fetal mortality. For every American newborn who dies, there are likely to be several who sustain neurological damage. Though it would be convenient to place the blame on socioeconomic factors or lack of hospital facilities, Haire argues that "modern" obstetrical practices are largely at fault. Evidence suggests that customs American women now take for granted, such as obstetrical medication, elective induction of labor, routine fetal heart monitoring, chemical stimulation of labor, and routine use of forceps, to mention only a few, not only distort the childbirth experience but can be damaging to the newborn.

In *Immaculate Deception,* Suzanne Arms argues that in order to control childbirth and make it more predictable, obstetricians devised a set of "interferences," which resulted in even greater but more predictable risk. More preventive technology was required "to interfere further with what was once a natural and uncomplicated process requiring no interference at all."[32]

Approximately 10 to 15 percent of deliveries pose a medical problem requiring intervention. In these cases modern obstetrical technology can be lifesaving. But there is increasing criticism of obstetrical practices that impose potentially damaging procedures on women who otherwise would experience a normal physiological event. Elective induction of labor is a classic example.

Under normal circumstances, oxytocin, a hormone released by the pituitary gland, stimulates the uterus to contract. Synthetic forms of the hormone are used by obstetricians to induce and to accelerate labor. Some induced labors are necessary because the well-being of the mother or the fetus requires a speedy termination of the pregnancy. However, during the late 1950s and early 1960s, elective induction, used to regulate the onset of labor, gained popularity, and the practice has increased steadily in many hospitals.[33] Obviously, induced childbirth is considerably more convenient for obstetricians, as one 1969 textbook honestly explains.

> There is universal agreement that the chief reason for electively inducing labor is to provide a more dependable schedule for the obstetrician. As Hall has said, ". . . it is high time we shed our shame over preferring to practice obstetrics in the daytime." If the safety of the gravida [pregnant woman] and her fetus can be assured, convenience for the obstetrician is a valid objective.[34]

However, obstetrical literature also documents a number of serious complications associated with elective inductions, including uterine spasm, fetal distress (too rapid, too slow, or irregular heartbeat of the fetus, or meconium staining — the premature release of fetal excrement), postpartum hemorrhage, prolapsed umbilical cord, premature separation of the placenta, and rupture of the uterus.[35]

The use of electronic fetal monitoring, a common practice in many United States hospitals, is another recent obstetrical intervention. It is designed to measure the fetal heart rate (FHR) against the stress of the mother's contractions. There is evidence to suggest that in addition to discomforting the laboring woman, who is immobilized by the apparatus, the monitoring may contribute to the distress it is designed to detect. Madeleine Shearer, editor of *Birth and the Family Journal,* notes that immobilization during labor may reduce placental blood flow and thus produce an abnormal FHR. When abnormal FHR is detected, such measures are taken as rolling the laboring woman on her side "often with a sense of gratitude that the monitor was able to pinpoint the alarm, rather than with the insight that the position and immobility of the mother might have been responsible for the emergency."[36]

There are two techniques for fetal monitoring: the external monitor, in which sensors are strapped by belts to the woman's abdomen, and the internal monitor, which produces a more precise measurement and consists of sensors and wires threaded through the vagina into the uterus and then attached to the fetal skull with a corresponding attachment on the uterus. To attach an internal monitor, artificial rupture of the amniotic sac, or bag of waters, is often necessary. Dr. Caldeyro-Barcía, past president of the International Federation of Gynecologists and Obstetricians and director of the Latin American Center for Perinatology and Human Development of the World Health Organization, has been an outspoken leader of the movement against obstetrical interferences. He argues that when the amniotic membranes have been ruptured, the protection of the fluid, which is important during contractions, is lost. Caldeyro-Barcía has shown that artificial rupture of the membranes can cause abnormal molding and compression of the fetal skull, as well as cord compression and labor that may be shortened below an optimum length of time.[37] Shearer adds that since high-risk fetuses are most vulnerable to head and cord compression, "we may wonder whether some of their abnormal FHR are due to the loss of protective fluid occasioned by internal monitoring."[38]

These hazards are acceptable when the risk of neonatal death is great. However, the most ambitious study to date of the effect of fetal monitoring on neonatal death presents data which suggest that in normal labor, with babies at term with no risk factor, the hazards of fetal monitoring may outweigh the risk of neonatal death. Analyzing data from 15,846 births at Beth Israel Hospital in Boston, the researchers conclude that the benefit from monitoring decreases as the inherent risk of the baby declines. In the highest risk group, 109 lives may be saved for every thousand babies monitored. But among babies at term with no risk factor, the neonatal death rate is approximately only one per thousand. "Even if fetal monitoring reduced their risk to zero, its absolute benefit could not exceed one life saved for every thousand babies monitored. Thus, the major effect of monitoring may be expected among the small group of infants whose risk is high enough to allow substantial reduction."[39]

Another development in obstetrics, undoubtedly linked to the frequent use of fetal monitoring, is the dramatic increase in the number of cesarean sections performed in the United States. Ironically, at the same time that movement is under way for a more natural, family-centered mode of childbirth, estimates are that as many as 25 percent of women now giving birth have cesarean sections.[40]

Traditionally, cesarean sections were performed for specific medical problems, such as cephalopelvic disproportion (a fetal head too large for the pelvic opening) or placenta previa (the placenta delivering before the fetus). Fetal distress, or distress detected by the fetal monitoring equipment, has been added to the list.

Current debate centers on the issue of whether many of these sections could have been avoided had obstetricians been more adept at distinguishing between real distress and the response of the baby to the normal stress of labor.[41] We may also wonder how many cesarean sections are done because of fetal distress caused by the use of the fetal monitoring equipment itself!

Obstetrical interventions have a place in complicated labors and deliveries, but consistent with the tradition established by nineteenth-century men-midwives and presaged by Elizabeth Nihell's attack on "meddlesome midwifery," aggressive intervention has become the custom in twentieth-century American obstetrics. To some observers it appears that obstetrics is on the verge of transforming childbirth into a totally surgical procedure.

Nineteenth-Century Pelvic Surgery

The emergence of modern gynecology is associated with nineteenth-century pelvic surgery in the United States. Obstetrics and gynecology were not yet officially wedded in one specialty during this century, but there was a connection between the two. Some gynecological techniques grew out of the trial-and-error efforts of "backwoods men-midwives" and their attempts to find remedies for obstetrical injuries. Nineteenth-century pelvic surgeons developed the majority of basic gynecological procedures and operations, with the exception of the hysterectomy. Eventually, pelvic surgery broadened into abdominal surgery, including the appendectomy, and renal, intestinal, and ureteral surgery. Gynecology broke away to form a specialty with emphasis on the female reproductive tract. Women, then, were the subjects on which abdominal surgery was first tried.

Medical history has been written from a perspective extremely sympathetic to physicians. The patient's role has been largely ignored, the issue of medical ethics has been vastly underplayed, and critical analyses are almost nonexistent. In a manner consistent with these practices, historians and biographers of the early gynecologists, often themselves members of the medical profession, glorify these surgeons for their courage and daring use of the knife.[42]

In contrast, Barker-Benfield describes the early gynecologists as ruthless and ambitious.[43] His work, though not heralded by the AMA, is a major contribution to medical history and shows how attitudes, emerging from Victorian standards, affected actions. Barker-Benfield presents the thesis that, unlike most professions, gynecology developed because of ulterior motives. He asserts that the development and proliferation of gynecological surgical procedures such as the clitoridectomy and ovariectomy were attempts to retaliate against and control women, who, under the impetus of the Industrial Revolution, were increasingly entering the work force and stimulating the growth of the women's rights movement.[44] Rather than humanitarian concerns, Barker-Benfield argues, "hostility toward women and competition among men were the conditions for the rise of gynecology."[45]

Although the motivation for nineteenth-century gynecological procedures is difficult to prove, the records left in medical journals and books do document, with amazing candor, medical practices that today would be considered maleficent. The records can be used to show how theories relevant to "female problems" were postulated on culturally patterned attitudes about the nature and purpose of women and how these beliefs provided the justification for some surgical practices. Many popular theories were not rational or scientific, but because gynecologists were (and still are) the uncontested medical experts, they were able to exert social control over women. Medical and surgical judgment, as these documents reveal, is influenced by personal and cultural values as well as by scientific proof. Significantly, the records also provide evidence that it was nineteenth-century gynecologists who promoted the concept of aggressive surgery and the idea that surgical intervention was appropriate as a first rather than as a last resort. In this respect, it will become apparent that the growth and development of surgery has been largely due to competition among surgeons to attain professional prominence and wealth through the discovery or refinement of a new treatment, technique, or instrument. History provides a valuable lesson on the dangers of a medical system in which the only constraint on physician behavior is professional self-regulation.

J. Marion Sims, "The Father of Gynecology"

Of all the nineteenth-century gynecological surgeons, J. Marion Sims is the most famous and celebrated. Called "the father of gynecology," his major achievements include the discovery of the technique for closing vesicovaginal fistula, the founding of the New York Women's Hospital, the invention of the Sims speculum and numerous other instruments, and a belief in cleanliness when other physicians found hygiene a joke. Sims's statue stands in New York's Central Park opposite the New York Academy of Medicine and on the Capitol grounds of South Carolina and Alabama. On Sims's death, a noted colleague said, "If I were called upon to name the three men who in the history of all times had done the most for their fellow men, I would say George Washington, William Jenner, and Marion Sims."[46]

Sims's obituary in the *Journal of the American Medical Association* concluded, "His memory the whole profession loves to honor, for by his genius and devotion to medical science and art he advanced it [gynecology] in its resources to relieve human suffering as much, if not more, than any man who has lived within this century."[47] In contrast, Barker-Benfield states, "His [Sims's] greatest general influence was to encourage an extremely active, adventurous policy of surgical interference with women's sexual organs."[48] Sims's archetypic career reveals much about nineteenth-century medical treatment of women and about the men who emulated him.

Marion Sims, a Southerner, began his career in 1835 as a general practitioner, avoiding female problems because "if there was anything I hated, it was investigating the organs of the female pelvis."[49] Sims's attitude, similar to that expressed by men-midwives, was shared by other physicians of the period. There was, for example, considerable controversy about the use of the vaginal speculum.[50] Many physicians found vaginal examinations a distasteful and distressing duty,[51] believed that the use of a speculum eroded the moral character of women, and thought women who sought such examination did so for sexual gratification. Robert Brudenell Carter, who is known for having developed the first psychiatric theory of repression, cautioned physicians in 1853:

> No one who has realized the amount of moral evil wrought in girls . . . whose prurient desires have been increased by Indian hemp and partially gratified by medical manipulations, can deny that remedy is worse than disease. I have . . . seen young unmarried women, of the middle class of society, reduced by the constant use of the speculum, to the mental and moral condition of prostitutes; seeking to give themselves the same indulgence by the practice of solitary vice; and asking every medical practitioner . . . to institute an examination of the sexual organs.[52]

Sims's dislike of the female pelvis turned into fascination as he became interested in the case of Anarcha, a local slave, who had developed a vesicovaginal fistula as the result of a prolonged labor and instrument damage sustained when he delivered her. There was no cure for vesicovaginal fistula. Realizing that slave women with this condition were viewed by many owners as economic burdens because they were good for neither breeding nor work, Sims discovered that slaves provided a readily available source of material for surgical experimentation. He guessed there were others in rural Alabama with the same condition and soon found that "plantation owners were delighted to hand over to him such unprofitable incurables and he soon had seven young negro women who were otherwise quite healthy collected in a little [backwoods] hospital he had specially built."[53] Slaves had no rights. When surgery was to be performed, the owner, not the slave, gave permission. Sims is reported to have purchased one woman, on whom he wanted to operate, when permission wasn't granted by her owner.[54]

Interestingly, in his autobiography Sims referred to his work on vesicovaginal fistula as experimentation, not surgery. From 1845 to 1849 he kept the seven women in his hospital. Without anesthesia, which wasn't in general use as yet, he performed repeated experiments on them in an attempt to find a way to close a fistula permanently. The operations were, in his own words, so painful that "none but a woman could have borne them."[55] He operated on Anarcha thirty times without anesthesia and the others with "comparable frequency." As each experiment failed, the women's conditions worsened and became more painful, though his attention to cleanliness kept them from dying of sepsis.

His pursuit of a surgical solution for the vesicovaginal fistula has been described as a monomania and Sims called a surgical "zealot." Colleagues praised his "courage" and "endurance," but the local community became critical. Rumors began to circulate "that it was a terrible thing for Sims to be allowed to keep on using human beings as experimental animals for his unproven surgical theories."[56] Reflecting on his lack of success, Sims stated:

> My repeated failures brought about a degree of anguish that I cannot now depict even if it were desirable. All my

> spare time was given to developing a single idea, the seemingly visionary one of curing this sad affliction, which not infrequently follows the law pronounced by an offended God when he said of women: "In sorrow and suffering shalt thou bring forth children."[57]

Sims also speculated on the degree of anguish endured by his patients and puzzled over their apparent willingness to submit to his experiments. White women, he stated, "seemed unable to bear the operation's pain and discomfort," and he theorized that stoicism was part of the "negro racial endowment." The explanation was simple. In addition to the fact that it would have done a slave little good to resist a white man's orders, during the four years they were contained in his hospital Sims fed and sheltered the women and gave them "tremendous quantities of opium." Opium was used as a buffer against pain and "to prevent any activity of the bowels which might endanger the success of an operation." As a result of the administration of opium, the women had "severe constipation," lasting up to five weeks; the tactic "nowadays . . . would be considered little short of murderous."[58] Apparently the women became addicted to opium and were able to ensure themselves a supply of the drug only by submitting to Sims's continued experiments.

In his thirtieth experiment on Anarcha, Sims perfected the long-sought technique for closing vesicovaginal fistula, which for him resulted in fame and professional prominence and for women relief from this obstetrical injury. But history tends to record success, not failure. There is no record of the number of slaves like Anarcha who, because they were unprofitable for owners to keep, were used in medical and surgical experiments.

Sims's personal values, his belief in extensive procreation, and in woman's primary purpose as motherhood, dictated the problems he chose to attack. He believed "that it was his duty as a physician . . . to enable his patients to have as many children as possible"[59] and that if a woman had enough "fortitude and endurance" he could remove any obstacle to conception. "Nothing, not even danger of death for the patient or of remorse and ostracism for the surgeon, was as important as the one great necessity of enabling childless women to emerge, rejoicing, from their tragic, barren state."[60] Sims's belief in the value of motherhood was shared by other physicians, and, although there were notable exceptions,[61] as late as the 1920s the medical profession resisted the efforts of Margaret Sanger and the American birth control movement[62] to disperse contraceptive information.* Novel theories were devised to discourage women from using any type of birth control. For example, writing in 1904, a professor of gynecology stated with authority that conjugal onanism (coitus interruptus) caused cancer. His theory reflected not only a desire to control female fertility but a belief in the mysterious power of semen.

> While briefly reciting the consequences entailed upon the woman by the practice of conjugal onanism, we reserved for special mention the frightful danger of cancer of the womb. We have high authority for the statement that this loathsome disease has this cause for its origin more frequently than any other. Indeed, if the constitutional proclivity to cancer exist in an individual, the practice of this vice is *almost sure to develop it.* If the ejection of the seminal fluid upon the mouth of the womb and within the vagina be necessary to the attainment of pleasure in the sexual act, as we have already stated, it is absolutely indispensible to safety. There is in this fluid a certain *specific property* which, as it were, remedies the otherwise dangerous condition in which the womb and vagina are placed by the venereal excitement. And this property is peculiar, outside of and beyond the mechanical effect already referred to; consequently nothing can be devised to take its place, and, consequently, whenever the genital function is not com-

* It is interesting to note that the importance placed on fertility has not diminished among twentieth-century physicians or childless women. The recent success with test-tube conception has led to the creation of one clinic in Virginia and will likely lead to others. Solving childlessness appears to be as much an obsession today as it was in Sims's era.

> pleted physiologically, direct injury results. [Emphasis mine.][63]

Sims is credited with developing several techniques for solving the perplexing problem of infertility. He reported visiting the bedrooms of some women who suffered from vaginismus (spasm of the vagina causing intercourse to be painful), where he would apply ether so that their husbands could impregnate them. A more common surgical technique, "splitting the mouth and neck of a contracted uterus . . . became a common practice for him, even though this subjected him to sharp criticism from some of his contemporaries, who protested that such 'meddlesome surgery' was fraught with great danger."[64] After he acquired a microscope, Sims realized that much of his surgery for infertility had been unnecessary: a low sperm count, not the uterus, had often been the problem.

Sims was plagued by chronic diarrhea. Believing a northern climate would improve his health, he moved his family to New York around 1851. However, New York physicians prevented him from practicing in their hospitals. To overcome the Northerner's hostility to Southerners, Sims determined to open his own hospital, one that would treat only female problems and would draw for its clientele the impoverished immigrant women who were flooding into New York City. He reasoned there was little difference between Southern slaves and poor Northern immigrants; by providing free services, he could obtain a steady supply of subjects for surgical experimentation. In May 1855, amid considerable resistance from the medical community, the New York Women's Hospital opened, the first of its kind in the United States.

It is impossible to gauge the amount of experimentation that took place at the New York Women's Hospital, but during his tenure there, Sims is credited with introducing the idea of aggressive surgery. "At the Women's Hospital this conception of surgery as nothing but a last-resort measure was radically revised. Insofar as gynecology was concerned, Marion Sims tended to look upon the knife not as the last weapon, but as the first. In espousing this viewpoint he sometimes brought himself into conflict with the distinguished members of his Consulting Medical Board, several of whom considered unduly reckless his suggestion for operating not only on cases of vesicovaginal fistula but also on diverse other diseases and malformations of the female reproductive system."[65] In 1874 he was asked to resign from the hospital by the Board of Lady Managers, which, due to Sims's frequent European absences, had changed in composition from earlier days, when board members had been hand-picked by him. The reasons given for requesting Sims's resignation included displeasure over the lack of patient privacy created by his policy of inviting a large number of physicians into the surgical suite to observe his operative technique and the continuing reports of dangerous experiments he was performing.

Sims countered that the resignation request was due to his controversial stand in favor of cancer surgery, which was opposed by the Board of Lady Managers. The response of his colleagues, who had long since accepted him into their medical circles, was interesting. In 1875, a few months after resigning from the Women's Hospital, Sims was elected president of the American Medical Association. "The delegates who voted unanimously to give him this honor made no secret of the fact that the 'great' gynecologist's stand in the hospital controversy was the major factor influencing their choice."[66] Also influential had been Sims's firm stand against lay intervention in medical issues.

By his death, in 1883, Sims's reputation and influence as the "evangelist of healing to women" was worldwide. His book, *Clinical Notes on Uterine Surgery,* influenced other surgeons to take an active policy of surgical interference. "It's vivid recitals of success along unconventional lines had emboldened them to try surgical experiments which otherwise they would not have had the courage to undertake."[67] Marion Sims was, as Barker-Benfield noted, an "architect of the vagina."[68]

It is interesting that Marion Sims's career continues to invite controversy. At the one hundred and first annual meeting of the American Gynecological Society, in April 1978, gynecologist Irwin H. Kaiser, in a paper entitled "Reappraisals of J. Marion Sims,"[69] took issue with Barker-Benfield for a "rampant revision of history" and for his interpretation of Sims "as an archetype of evil masquerading as good." Kaiser's criticisms of Barker-Benfield are reasoned and thoughtful. Noting that women with fistulas became social outcasts, he argues that the injury was a major social problem to women who sustained them. Thus, though Kaiser agrees that it is proper to criticize Sims for "excessive zeal in perfecting fistula repair," he also argues that Sims's "eventual success is a tribute to his ingenuity and skill as well as to his astounding pertinacity."

Kaiser points out that Barker-Benfield has applied the social standards of 1975 to decisions and conduct that took place in 1850. Kaiser concludes:

> One might more appropriately deplore slavery and the low status of women in 1850 and Sims' insensitivity to them. The criticisms are therefore not devoid of merit. Sims did develop his vesicovaginal fistula repair by multiple procedures on slaves and immigrants, and he did this before the availability of anesthetics. It is difficult to envisage today the desperate status of an 1850 woman with total urinary incontinence, and it is against this background that evaluation must be made. It is not easy to decide whether Sims acted out of callousness or compassion. It is certain that he used his patients, an act perhaps mitigated by their own active participation in the search for a cure . . . Sims was the product of his times: insensitive and ingenious, difficult and dedicated, a physician whose medical accomplishments have borne up well in the test of time.[70]

Official reaction to Kaiser's paper was negative. Sims's supporters appear unable to bear any criticism of the man they exalt as their leader. For example, claiming that Kaiser had "hinted that J. Marion Sims, the father of American gynecology, and a former President of this Society, may not have been the upstanding gentleman that we have all accepted him to be, but rather a white racist and male chauvinist to boot," Denis Cavanagh, a Florida gynecologist concluded:

> Lest this distinguished Society degenerate into just another social club, we all have a responsibility to supply the program committee with good scientific papers. In my opinion this paper damns Sims with faint praise and is one of the least impressive papers that I have heard before this Society. Indeed, just about the only thing on which I can congratulate the author is the neatly typed manuscript.[71]

Sims wasn't the only vaginal architect at work, nor was experimentation limited to fistula repair. Especially controversial was the widespread practice of female castration or ovariectomy, an operation whose history has been called the history of pelvic surgery.

Female Castration — The Ovariectomy

Though little has been written about Kentuckian Ephraim McDowell, called the "father of ovariectomy," he performed the first preanesthesia female castration in 1809 in his backwoods home. It is Robert Battey, however, who is credited with popularizing the technique for removing female ovaries. Discussing the profound influence of Battey's invention, George Engelmann, president of the American Gynecological Society in 1900, stated, "Robert Battey led the advance onward; he taught us that organs could be removed with impunity, and from the ovariectomy and salpingotomy [incision of a Fallopian tube] the knife has successfully attacked every part within the abdominal cavity, until even the diaphragm no longer limits its progress."[72]

Barker-Benfield states that popularity of the ovariectomy peaked between 1880 and 1900 but that it was still performed for psychological disorders as late as 1946.[73] During the period of popularity, female castration was used to treat a number of problems. In addition to suspected cases of ovarian disease, "normal ovariectomy" was performed for epilepsy, nymphomania, and especially for nervous and psychological problems such as hysteria and "ovarian insanity."

A connection between the female sexual organs and insanity has a tradition dating to Hippocrates, in the fifth and fourth centuries B.C.[74] Barbara Ehrenreich and Deirdre English refer to it as the "psychology of the ovary," a widely held belief that "woman's entire personality was directed by the ovaries, and any abnormalities, from irritability to insanity, could be traced to some ovarian disease."[75] They point out that the rationale for the operation flowed from the theory. Psychological disorders were a sign of ovarian disease because the ovaries controlled personality.[76] Typical of this belief, an 1883 book entitled *Perils of American Women, or, a Doctor's Talk with Maiden, Wife, and Mother* carried the following message: "Suffice it to say, briefly, that any inflammatory affliction of the ovaries, any displacement, produces most marked effects upon the brain and nervous system. Thus we see indigestion, spinal irritation, many forms of neuralgia, headaches, mental irritability, and insanity, all largely attributable to some disease of the ovaries."[77] Pelvic surgeons contributed their unique solution, female castration.

In 1881, reflecting on the state of gynecology, James Chadwick outlined the pattern of development through which many "have sought to attain immortality by propounding new theories, devising new operations, and, above all, by inventing new instruments."[78] New operations, he explained, had a predictable life history. An article in a medical journal would describe the success obtained by the author in the treatment of a certain condition by a new operative method. Immediately, the technique would be tried by many practitioners, who would also publish their results, "particularly if favorable, when they may expect to derive renown or practice from being early identified with the innovation."[79] As a consequence, negative outcomes were less likely to be known, and the only barrier to experimentation was the ethical position of individual surgeons.

Eventually, negative or unfavorable results began to be published, and the operation was either adopted as a regular surgical procedure or forgotten.

The ovariectomy followed a similar pattern. In the twenty years that it was popular among gynecologists as a treatment for nervous disorders, numerous articles in support of the operation were published in medical journals. For example, in 1882 a professor of clinical gynecology at the University of Pennsylvania wrote:

> The disorders of menstrual life, for which the ovaries have been successfully removed, are fibroid tumors of the womb, chronic pelvic peritonitis, persistent ovaritis [inflamed ovaries] and ovaralgia [ovarian pain], ovarian epilepsy, dysmenorrhea, menorrhagia . . . to this list there can be no doubt that some forms of insanity ought to be added. The relation which they bear to menstruation is often a very close one — so close indeed that the term, ovarian insanity, would best define it . . . Since the verdict of the profession is largely in favor of the removal of the ovaries for many physical derangements dependent upon menstruation, the same remedy should *a fortiori* be tried for those mental derangements which plainly arise or seem to arise from the same source. The objections to such remedy when applied for mental diseases, are in fact less valid than when it is resorted to for physical lesions. For, in the first place, an insane woman is no more a member of the body-politic, than a criminal; secondly, her death is always a relief to her dearest friends; thirdly, even in case of her recovery from mental disease, she is liable to transmit the taint of insanity to her children and to her children's children for many generations. The removal, therefore, of the ovaries in such a case, would tend to restore a woman to home and to society, and it would at the same time effectively bar her from having an insane offspring.[80]

Part of the argument for castration was related to the idea that insanity was inherited, but an equally important function of the procedure was the social and sexual control of women. Case histories published in medical journals revealed that husbands sometimes ordered their wives' castration when duties were not performed to satisfaction. Barker-Benfield observes that "disorderly women were handed over to the gynecologist for castration and other kinds of radical treatment by husbands or fathers unable to enforce their minimum identity guarantee — the submission of women."[81] In 1896, Dr. David Gilliam made it clear that he believed castration made women obedient and argued for greater use of the ovariectomy.

> Rohé, Manton, and others have blazed the way; and what do they tell us? They tell us castration pays; that patients are improved, some of them cured; that the moral sense of the patient is elevated, that she becomes tractable, orderly, industrious, and cleanly . . . My own experience in this line has been most happy.[82]

The ovariectomy had critics, and in time unfavorable articles were published in medical journals. In 1886 a pathologist charged that gynecologists were allowing their enthusiasm for surgery to influence their idea of ovarian pathology.[83] Through case histories, others demonstrated that epilepsy and insanity were rarely improved by castration. One perceptive critic told colleagues that in the few cases where improvement was noted, it was due to "the profound impression upon the mind of the subject rather than upon the removal of the ovaries," and he cautioned gynecologists about the possible legal ramifications of the practice. "What the medico-legal complications are that may arise in the future from the wholesale unsexing of women that has gone on in recent years it is difficult to predict."[84]

The gynecologists' attack on the ovary serves to illustrate an important point. Because nineteenth-century women trusted their gynecologists' "expert" advice, they were convinced that their problems were personal and ovarian and that surgery was the miracle cure.[85] When gynecologists stated with authority that an ovariectomy solved female problems, some women willingly sought relief through castration. Twentieth-century women, like their Victorian sisters, still, often uncritically, accept the gynecologist's expert advice. Every year thousands of women are convinced that a hysterectomy and sometimes an accompanying castration will improve their health. Likewise, many women are persuaded that childbirth is a medical problem that can be resolved best through the use of unnatural interferences. In his 1906 address to the American Gynecological Society, Ely Van De Warker delivered a message as pertinent today as it was then.

> The sociological relations of the mistakes about the ovaries have been brought into the daily life of the woman. So constantly have they been held up before her as the one evil spot in her anatomy, that she has grown to look with suspicion upon her own organs. Neither the patient nor the average doctor thinks sanely on this subject . . . The woman appears to give the value to her ovaries that the doctor does to the danger of the operation. [Van De Warker believed there was little or no danger.] The result is that we have an overwilling surgeon and a pliant patient.[86]

The Clitoridectomy, a Cure for Masturbators

Nineteenth-century surgeons were also perplexed by woman's sexuality. Nymphomania and related types of so-called insanity were believed caused by masturbation. Some physicians recommended castration; others discovered that removal of the clitoris, the female organ responsible for sexual sensation and arousal, eliminated the problem.

For the invention of the clitoridectomy, history is indebted to "a successful London ovariotomist," Baker-Brown, who was alleged to suffer from "extensive cerebral softening," which affected his judgment. "He found that a number of 'semi-demented' epileptics were habitual masturbators, and that the masturbation was, in women, chiefly effected by excitement of the mucous membrane on and around the clitoris."[87] Before he was censured by the "Commissioner of Lunacy" and expelled from the London Obstetrical Society, Baker-Brown "operated on an enormous number of cases." Baker-Brown was wrong about the connection with epilepsy, but he was accurate about the locus of female sexual feeling and, as other physicians learned, had discovered an effective method of controlling female sexual activity.

Gynecologists were not the first to suggest that masturbation had dire consequences. Thomas Szasz[88] cites the case of "masturbation madness" to illustrate how psychiatry manufactured mental illness. During the nineteenth century, masturbation, or, as it was also called, onanism or self-abuse, was believed to cause numerous physical disorders that could result in death as well as dementia and overall moral decay. Individuals who practiced this "solitary vice" were viewed as criminals and the act itself as a crime.

Attitudes about female masturbation were linked, in part, to beliefs about appropriate female sexual behavior. In contrast to the uncontrollable sexual urges of men, women were supposed to be sexually passive. Since impregnation can occur without female arousal, men reasoned that women should be relatively passionless. For example, in his 1888 article on masturbation, Lawson Tait, a noted surgeon and gynecologist, stated:

> The female organism has always been merely the vehicle for the maturation of the ovum, and for the receptacle of the fertilizing influence of the male; being, in fact, what we may call the passive factor in the reproductive act. For her part in the process, then, only enough of sexual passion or instinct is required to indicate to the male the stage at which his share may be effectively performed. For the male, on the contrary, a constant tendency to aggression is necessary, that he may be in readiness at the time required . . . Through countless generations of all animals, the sexual instinct, above all others, has been developed in the males by the constant elimination of the least fit, and the subsequent success of the sexually fittest . . . It

> ought to be, therefore, no matter of surprise that in the human race the sexual instinct is very powerful in man, and comparatively weak in women.[89]

Though masturbation was thought to be less frequent among females than among males, it was still strongly condemned; it violated the notion that women were passive, passionless sexual beings. Both male and female violators were punished. Szasz writes that an English physician recommended male masturbators wear locked chastity belts by day, and spiked or toothed rings by night, the latter to awaken them in the case of a nocturnal erection. Another physician recommended circumcision for prevention and treatment. Among women the "moral leprosy" was treated surgically, and Szasz notes that clitoridectomy was advocated for this purpose until the turn of the century.[91] With surgical tools, gynecologists, in effect, enforced moral values and in so doing stepped beyond the legitimate bounds of their professional expertise and became the final arbitrators of virtue and sin.[91]

The 1901 "Transactions of the Women's Hospital Society" describes several cases of masturbation "cured" by Dr. W. Gill Wylie, Marion Sims's medical partner and staff member of the New York Women's Hospital. For example:

> A year ago Dr. Wylie saw a young Jewess. She had a history of painful menstruation and other symptoms of some local trouble. She had grown very nervous, became very much deranged, and had not spoken a word for two years. Everything about her indicated that she was insane. She apparently understood conversation, although she would not speak. Examination revealed positive evidence of masturbation, the clitoris being enlarged. The uterus was dilated and curetted, a drainage tube introduced, and later the clitoris was amputated. She generally improved in health and was not caught masturbating, for some time at any rate, and she began to walk about, but she would not speak. She was sent to the country with an ordinary

> nurse. She played on the piano and gained in physical health, and returned in four months in a most perfect physical condition . . . After being watched closely, with no signs of again attempting to masturbate, and not showing any positive amorous signs, she was considered about cured.[92]

No doubt the overwhelming disapproval of the "experts" created a strong sense of guilt in many women who used masturbation as an outlet for sexual tension, and many must have been convinced by their physicians that they were, in fact, depraved for doing so.

There are no statistics to gauge accurately the prevalence of clitoridectomy, but Barker-Benfield states that, although it was never as popular a surgical procedure in the United States as ovariectomy, it coexisted with and then was superseded by female circumcision. "Both clitoridectomy and circumcision aimed to check what was thought to be a growing incidence of female masturbation, an activity which men feared inevitably aroused women's naturally boundless but usually repressed sexual appetite for men."[93] By 1920, clitoridectomy and normal ovariectomy for epilepsy, insanity, and nymphomania had decreased in popularity, and eventually gynecologists dropped them from their surgical repertoire. The ovariectomy remained a procedure for surgical removal of diseased ovaries but surfaced again, along with the hysterectomy, as a gynecological remedy for cancer prevention and permanent sterilization. It is Barker-Benfield's thesis that today the hysterectomy and mastectomy have replaced female castration as vehicles for male aggression.[94]

The history of obstetrics appears more benign than that of gynecology because much of the operative experimentation by men-midwives was directed at solving the very real problems of dangerous and painful childbirth. Gynecologists, on the other hand, used surgery to enforce values and control women, and, too, many were ambitious, competitive men who sought professional prominence and wealth by manipulation and excavation of the female pelvis. But there was a commonality beyond professional interest in the reproductive organs. Obstetricians, like gynecologists, favored aggressive, surgical intervention, an orientation that carried into the twentieth century. George Engelmann's 1900 presidential speech before the American Gynecological Society summarized the century's surgical innovations and predicted events to come.

> We seem to have attained the apex of surgical achievement but there are peaks beyond, new fields to conquer . . . We cannot with safety rest on past achievements; we must struggle onward . . . The task before us now is that we reduce morbidity as we have mortality; now that we can with impunity remove organs, we must endeavor to preserve and to restore healthy functional activity. I can but quote one of our progressive surgeons, who well said that in the last twenty-five years we have come from the fear of handling the pelvis to the fear of not removing some part of its contents; from the dread of interference of any kind to the fearless taking out of any and every organ . . . Along the lines of extirpation we can no longer advance; we must look to preservation, to the conserving of the function, and this I believe to be the surgery of the twentieth century. Experiment must pave the way if progress is to continue, and though mistakes will at first be made, we must persevere.[95]

Twentieth Century: Primary Care Physician or Superspecialist?

By the turn of the twentieth century, a number of physicians had become interested in both branches of the female specialty and thought it made little sense to base two distinct and separate specialties on one anatomic region of one sex. In 1920, the American Board of Obstetrics and Gynecology incorporated, cementing the union of obstetrics and gynecology in the United States.[96]

Within the medical profession, twentieth-century obstetrics and gynecology suffers a tarnished image. The status and glamour of the specialty have waned since the early days, when pelvic surgeons were exalted as noble pathfinders, blazing the surgical trail. The new surgical trailblazers are experimentalists, such as heart surgeons; in contrast, obstetrics and gynecology appears routine, with limited potential for surgical expansion.

One writer believes this image, reflected in the attitude of medical students, views obstetricians and gynecologists as "skilled laborers" performing the duties of "baby catchers" and "uterus snatchers." He attributes it to the declining birthrate and to the inability of the public to understand the importance of the preventive medicine delivered by the profession as well as a failure to see it as a research-oriented discipline.[97]

Obstetrician-gynecologists are looked on by members of other branches of medicine as substandard surgeons whose ability beyond cesarean section and simple hysterectomy is inadequate. The reputation of gynecologists as incompetent surgeons is pervasive enough that some hospitals restrict gynecologists' privileges to simple gynecological procedures, requesting that they not attempt repairs of injuries to surrounding tissues.[98]

Reducing the challenge of gynecology further, in most areas of the United States gynecology lost breast surgery to general surgery; the younger gynecological surgeons today no longer have the skill to perform mastectomies and related types of operations. General surgery is not the only field encroaching on and posing a threat to obstetrics and gynecology. In a display of medical imperialism, the president of the Central Association of Obstetricians and Gynecologists summed up, in 1973, the problem in an unflattering allegory.

> Today I propose to explore with you the status of our semiprivate preserve — the pelvic pool, and our members-only fishermen's club — Gynecology and Obstetrics . . . Originially there were only three organizations concerned with body ecology. One group devoted to all things botanical — medicine, a second concerned with wild life management — surgery, and finally the propagation

> group — Obstetrics and Gynecology . . . As time passed the botanical and wild life management groups have subdivided in accordance with the increased knowledge and specialized interests of members. Easements in our club property have been granted to the newer colon surgery and urology clubs. Silting of our ponds has occurred as a result of activities of the botanists and their affiliates. In turn we have built high fences to prevent further intrusions . . . Our contacts with other groups have been limited. We have suffered from inbreeding and seemingly are threatened on all sides. It is imperative that something be done before further silting, overgrowth, more land grabs, and poaching result in total disintegration of our historically important club.[99]

Added to the problems of the specialty is the move by some medical schools to reduce obstetrics and gynecology to an elective subject, thus suggesting to the medical student that the field is unnecessary to the completion of the core curriculum on which a medical degree is based.

The lack of prestige of obstetrics and gynecology, depicted as boring work, limited in scope and involving long hours, and the declining importance placed on the specialty in medical schools resulted in recruitment problems for the profession. This meant that many candidates were drawn from low achievers in medical school classes[100] and from foreign medical school graduates.[101]

The problems faced by the field were threatening enough to some members to move the 1969 president of the New York Obstetrical Society to state:

> Obstetrics and gynecology is in trouble, deep trouble . . . because of our inability to establish obstetrics and gynecology as one of the major disciplines beyond dispute in the area not only of medicine but also of health . . . We are approaching a time of very considerable peril for our discipline. At this time we are still fighting frontier skirmishes with surgeons, who have suggested that training

> in gynecology be preceded with a two-year residency in general; with pediatricians, who have long outstripped us in research and training grants, and who are now developing keen interests in the intrauterine fetus, not to speak of family planning for the adolescent and young mother; and most of all with deans, who across the country are cutting into obstetric teaching time and seem determined to make obstetrics a paramedical public health problem.[102]

Efforts to improve the position of obstetrics and gynecology within medicine, and to encourage more and better American medical students to enter the specialty, have been centered primarily on two tactics. Attempts have been made to portray obstetrics and gynecology as a desirable career by emphasizing research, promoting group practice in obstetrics, and, especially, by developing more attractive training programs. Coincidental with these efforts, new interest in the use of trained nurse-midwives has been growing within the medical community. Interest on the part of some health workers indicates concern about the continued high infant-mortality rates in the United States. But among many obstetrician-gynecologists, reintroduction of midwives appears to be motivated by other factors. One study found that obstetricians consider nurse-midwives able to perform those jobs that require a combination of the most time and least skill and unable to perform "skilled or professional functions."[103] The president of the American Association of Obstetricians and Gynecologists in a 1972 address stressed the importance of the use of midwives to make obstetrics more attractive to the students who are "turned off when they see respected specialists delivering their own patients at 2:00 A.M."[104]

Other attempts to improve the image of the profession are more controversial. Disagreement over the emphasis and direction of the specialty is noted in the professional journals and has resulted in a certain amount of intraprofessional fighting.

During a 1969 conference on specialization convened by the American Board of Obstetricians and Gynecologists, three ad hoc committees were appointed to consider subspecialization in gynecologic oncology, fetal and maternal medicine, and gynecologic endocrinology and infertility. In 1973, the ABOG was authorized by the American Board of Medical Specialists to certify through examination "superspecialists" in these three areas. The ABOG stated that "this is a development solely for improving and then recognizing an obstetrician-gynecologist's ability to deal with more complicated problems."[105] The result of this move was to sharpen the lines between competing segments within the profession.

The effect of the superspecialist is hotly debated by the practitioners in the field, many of whom believe that it will result in the fragmentation of the specialty and reduce the work of the nonspecialist to the most routine level. Many practitioners believe the emphasis should be placed on promoting the obstetrican-gynecologist as the primary care physician of women. They present convincing evidence that this is the role most commonly performed by contemporary practitioners of the specialty.[106]

Obstetrics and gynecology is a specialty in flux, beset with internal and external conflict and plagued by low esteem. The strategy of encroaching on other medical and surgical specialties (oncology, endocrinology, and pediatrics) has been undertaken in an effort to make the specialty more attractive and to survive medical imperialism and the conflict over body territory. These conditions within the profession, combined with the traditional emphasis on aggressive intervention in childbirth and on the organs of reproduction, create a climate ripe for exploitative practices and helps to explain today's soaring rates of gynecological surgery. The interplay of these factors can be seen in the training of new practitioners.

Notes

1. Margaret Mead and Niles Newton, "Cultural Patterning of Perinatal Behavior," in *Childbearing — Its Social and Psychological Aspects,* Stephen Richardson and Alan Guttmacher, eds. (Baltimore: The Williams and Wilkins Company, 1967.)

2. For instance, women can give birth in a variety of positions. In the United States, where childbirth is treated as a surgical procedure, women are placed in the lithotomy position, with back flat and legs up, despite the fact that woman's ability to push is significantly reduced in the lithotomy position. In the majority of non-European societies for which there is information, an upright position, either kneeling or sitting, is most common. Many cultures use pushing, pulling, and bracing devices. In some societies, like the Aranda of central Australia, women squat and are assisted by two female attendants, one in front to catch the baby and one in back to support the mother-to-be on her lap. See Michael Newton and Niles Newton, "The Propped Position for the Second Stage of Labor," *Obstetrics and Gynecology* 15 (1960), and Mead and Newton, "Cultural Patterning," p. 218.
3. For a history of midwives and other women healers, see Barbara Ehrenreich and Deirdre English, *Witches, Midwives, and Nurses* (Oyster Bay, New York: Glass Mountain Pamphlets).
4. Samuel Gregory, "Man-Midwifery Exposed and Corrected" (1848), in *The Male Mid-Wife and the Female Doctor: The Gynecology Controversy in Nineteenth Century America,* Charles Rosenberg and Carroll Smith-Rosenberg, eds. (New York: Arno Press, 1974), p. 9.
5. Richard Wertz and Dorothy Wertz, *Lying-In: A History of Childbirth in America* (New York: The Free Press, 1977).
6. The Wertzes point out that the prohibition against exposure of the female retarded clinical training in obstetrics. They relate the incidents surrounding the first use of a woman for instructional purposes. Before this, students were not allowed to observe deliveries; their training came entirely from reading books. In 1850, Dr. James White of Buffalo, apparently believing he had found a solution, demonstrated a live birth with a poor Irish immigrant woman pregnant with her second illegitimate child, because "doctors could classify such women as not needing or deserving the same symptomatic treatment given to respectable women." Twenty men observed for five minutes, long enough to prompt a local physician to write in the town paper that the students had become sexually aroused. The case came to the attention of the American Medical Association, which "deprecated the exposure of a patient during delivery as unnecessary since a physician had to learn to conduct labor by touch alone or he was unfit to practice." Though some physicians favored the improved medical training such exposure of women would permit, others feared that if men couldn't perform obstetrical operations without seeing what they were doing, women would be so offended that male midwives would lose out to female midwives.
7. Gregory, "Man-Midwifery Exposed," p. 1.

8. Ibid., p. 12.
9. Though it is a popular belief that Julius Caesar was delivered in this manner and that the cesarean section was named for him, many scholars now disagree. Caesar's mother lived for many years after his birth, a feat that would have been virtually impossible, since in those days the operation was always fatal. More likely, the name derives from the Latin word "to cut," or from the mandate of the emperors, or Caesars, that postmortem sections be performed on women who died late in pregnancy. See Harold Speert, *Iconographia Gyniatrica: A Pictorial History of Gynecology and Obstetrics* (Philadelphia: F. A. Davis Company, 1973), pp. 297–302.
10. Gregory, "Man-Midwifery Exposed," p. 29.
11. Harvey Graham and Isaac Flack, *Eternal Eve: The Mysteries of Birth and the Customs That Surround It* (London: Hutchinson Press, 1960), p. 123.
12. Ibid., p. 158.
13. Wertz and Wertz, *Lying-In*, p. 37.
14. Gregory, "Man-Midwifery Exposed," p. 29.
15. Ibid., p. 32.
16. William Myers, "The Limitations of Craniotomy," *Transactions of the American Association of Obstetrics and Gynecology*, 8 (1895).
17. A. M. Mauriceau, "The Married Woman's Private Medical Companion" (1847), in *Sex, Marriage and Society*, Charles Rosenberg and Carroll Smith-Rosenberg, eds. (New York: Arno Press, 1974), pp. 188–189.
18. Graham and Flack, *Eternal Eve*, p. 213.
19. Frances Kobrin, "The American Midwife Controversy: A Crisis of Professionalization," *Bulletin of the History of Medicine* 40 (1966) 350.
20. J. Clifton Edgar, "The Remedy for the Midwife Problem," *American Journal of Obstetrics*, 63 (1911), 882.
21. Kobrin, "American Midwife Controversy," p. 351.
22. J. Whitridge Williams, "Medical Education and the Midwife Problem in the United States," *The Journal of the American Medical Association*, 58 (1912), 1.
23. Ibid., p. 7.
24. Clara Noyes, "Training of Midwives in Relation to the Prevention of Infant Mortality," *American Journal of Obstetrics*, 66 (1912), 1056.
25. Arthur Emmons and James Huntingdon, "The Midwife: Her Future in the United States," *American Journal of Obstetrics* 65 (1912), 394.
26. Abraham Flexner, *Medical Education in the United States and Canada: A Report to the Carnegie Foundation for the Advancement of Teaching* (New York: Carnegie Foundation, 1910).
27. Kobrin, "American Midwife Controversy," p. 357.
28. Ibid., p. 359.

29. Beatrice Mongeau, Harvey Smith, and Ann Maney, "The 'Granny' Midwife: Changing Roles and Functions of a Folk Practitioner," *American Journal of Sociology,* 66 (1960).
30. G. J. Barker-Benfield, *The Horrors of the Half-Known Life* (New York: Harper and Row, 1976).
31. Doris Haire, *The Cultural Warping of Childbirth* (Rochester, New York: International Childbirth Education Association, 1972).
32. Suzanne Arms, *Immaculate Deception* (Boston: Houghton Mifflin, 1975), p. 53.
33. Luis Cibils, "Enhancement and Induction of Labor," in *Risks in the Practice of Modern Obstetrics,* Silvio Aladjem, ed. (St. Louis: C. V. Mosby, 1975), p. 193.
34. Kenneth Niswander, "Elective Induction of Labor," in *Controversies in Obstetrics and Gynecology,* Duncan Reid and T. C. Barton, eds. (Philadelphia: W. B. Saunders, 1969), p. 122.
35. See Roberto Caldeyro-Barcía, "Some Consequences of Obstetrical Interference," *Birth and the Family Journal,* 2 (1975), 34–38; Harry Fields, "Complications of Elective Induction," *Obstetrics and Gynecology,* 15 (1960), 476–80.
36. Madeleine Shearer, "Some Deterrents to Objective Evaluation of Fetal Monitors," *Birth and the Family Journal,* 2 (1975), 58.
37. Caldeyro-Barcía, "Some Consequences," pp. 34–38.
38. Shearer, "Some Deterrents," p. 58.
39. Raymond Neutra, Stephen Fienberg, Sander Greenland, and Emanuel Friedman, "Effect of Fetal Monitoring on Neonatal Death Rates," *The New England Journal of Medicine,* 299 (1978), 3.
40. "Women and Health Roundtable Report," 2 (1978), 3.
41. Deborah Larned, "Cesarean Births: Why They are Up 100 Percent," *Ms.* magazine, October 1978.
42. Graham and Flack, *Eternal Eve,* p. 268.
43. Barker-Benfield, *Horrors.*
44. G. J. Barker-Benfield, "The Spermatic Economy: A Nineteenth Century View of Sexuality," *Journal of Feminist Studies,* 1 (1972), 45–74.
45. Barker-Benfield, *Horrors,* p. 96.
46. Seale Harris, *Woman's Surgeon* (New York: Macmillan Company, 1950), p. 373.
47. Ibid.
48. Barker-Benfield, *Horrors,* p. 91.
49. J. Marion Sims, *The Story of My Life* (New York: D. Appleton and Company, 1889), p. 231.
50. Graham and Flack, *Eternal Eve,* p. 259.
51. C. D. Meigs, "Females and their Diseases, A Series of Letters to his Classes" (1848), quoted in Milton Abramson. "Preparation for Marriage and Parenthood," in *Psychosomatic Obstetrics, Gynecology,*

and Endocrinology, William S. Kroger, ed. (Springfield: C. Thomas, Publisher, 1962), p. 169.

52. Robert Brudenell Carter, *On the Pathology and Treatment of Hysteria* (London: John Churchill, 1853), p. 69.
53. Graham and Flack, *Eternal Eve,* p. 237.
54. Richard Shryack, *Medicine in America* (Baltimore: Johns Hopkins Press, 1966), p. 167.
55. Graham and Flack, *Eternal Eve,* p. 237.
56. Harris, *Woman's Surgeon,* p. 99.
57. Graham and Flack, *Eternal Eve,* p. 237.
58. Harris, *Woman's Surgeon,* p. 100.
59. Ibid., p. 48.
60. Ibid., p. 184.
61. See Mauriceau, "Private Medical Companion."
62. See David Kennedy, *Birth Control in America* (New Haven: Yale University Press, 1970); Margaret Sanger, *Margaret Sanger: An Autobiography* (New York: Dover Publications, 1971).
63. William Wallings, *Sexology* (Philadelphia: Puritan Publishing Company, 1904), pp. 72–73 (Arno Press Reprint Series, *Sex, Marriage and Society,* 1974).
64. Harris, *Woman's Surgeon,* p. 180.
65. Ibid., p. 160.
66. Ibid., p. 308.
67. Ibid., p. 268.
68. Barker-Benfield, *Horrors,* p. 91.
69. Irwin H. Kaiser, "Reappraisals of J. Marion Sims," *American Journal of Obstetrics and Gynecology,* 132 (1978), 878–884.
70. Kaiser, "Reappraisals," pp. 881–882.
71. Ibid., pp. 882–883.
72. George Engelmann, "The American Girl of Today," *American Journal of Obstetrics,* 42 (1900), 755.
73. Barker-Benfield, *Horrors,* p. 121.
74. See Pauline Bart and Diana Scully, "The Politics of Hysteria: The Case of the Wandering Womb," in *Gender and Disordered Behavior: Sex Differences in Psychopathology,* Edith Gomberg and Violet Franks, eds. (Larchmont, New York: Bruner/Mazel, 1979).
75. Barbara Ehrenreich and Deirdre English, *For Her Own Good: 150 Years of the Expert's Advice to Women* (New York: Anchor Press/Doubleday, 1978), p. 109.
76. Ibid., p. 112.
77. George Austin, *Perils of American Women, or, a Doctors Talk with Maiden, Wife, and Mother* (Boston: Lee and Shepard, 1883), quoted in *Roots of Bitterness,* Nancy Cott, ed. (New York: E. P. Dutton and Company, 1972), p. 296.

78. James Chadwick, "Obstetric and Gynecologic Literature, 1876–1881," *Transactions of the American Medical Association,* 32 (1881), 254.
79. Ibid.
80. William Goodell, "Clinical Notes on the Extirpation of the Ovaries for Insanity," *American Journal of Insanity,* 38 (1882), 294–295.
81. Barker-Benfield, *Horrors,* pp. 129–130.
82. David Gilliam, "Oophorectomy for the Insanity and Epilepsy of the Female: A Plea for Its More General Adoption," *Transactions of the American Association of Obstetricians and Gynecologists,* 9 (1896), 320.
83. Henry Coe, "Is Disease of the Uterine Appendages as Frequent as it Has Been Represented?" *American Journal of Obstetrics* 19 (1886), 561–575.
84. Allan Hamilton, "The Abuse of Oophorectomy in Diseases of the Nervous System," *New York Medical Journal,* 57 (1893), 182.
85. For a discussion of the history of expert's advice to women, see Ehrenreich and English, *For Her Own Good.* For a discussion of hysterical illness in nineteenth-century women, see Carroll Smith-Rosenberg, "The Hysterical Woman: Sex Roles and Role Conflict in 19th Century America," *Social Research,* 39 (1972), 652–678.
86. Ely Van De Warker, "The Fetch of the Ovary," *American Journal of Obstetrics,* 54 (1906), 372.
87. Lawson Tait, "Masturbation," *The Medical News* 53 (1888), 2.
88. Thomas Szasz, *The Manufacture of Madness* (Australia: Paladin, 1973).
89. Tait, "Masturbation," p. 1.
90. Szasz, *Manufacture,* p. 221.
91. It is interesting to note that the social definition of the sexual nature of women has changed over the past one hundred years. Victorian women were supposed to be passionless, and their interest in sex was considered abnormal. In line with this view, nineteenth-century pelvic surgery often robbed women of their sexuality. In contrast, the modern twentieth-century woman is more likely to be viewed as abnormal if she is uninterested in sex or unable to achieve her expected multiorgasmic potential. Consistent with this view, James C. Burt, a gynecologist in Dayton, Ohio, has designed a surgical procedure that he calls love surgery, and that, he alleges, increases women's orgasmic potential. As Burt sees it, women are prevented from being totally orgasmic because the anatomical design of the female vagina is faulty. He argues that the clitoris is not accessible enough to penile stimulation during intercourse, thus causing "structural coital inadequacy in the human female." To compensate for this, Burt has designed an operation that critics term "The Mark II Vagina." For about

$1500, women can purchase the Mark II which consists of lengthening the existing vagina by severing the pubococcygeal muscle to create an alien set of female genitalia in which the vaginal opening, smaller, has been moved closer to the clitoris.

Besides the obvious sexist implications of the surgery, the procedure is considered by critics to be hazardous. Dr. Diane S. Fordney, Associate Professor of Gynecology at the State University of New York at Stony Brook, calls the reconstruction "totally anatomically inappropriate" and points out that the pubococcygeal muscle gives partial support to the bladder. Its severing may result in a significant risk of urinary prolapse. Furthermore, the operation carries all the usual traumata of major surgery, including death by anesthesia. And because Burt's follow-up procedures appear to be unsystematic, there may be no real proof that the Mark II accomplishes its inventor's claim. Burt used to offer the reconstruction to women who were having other types of vaginal surgery, including episiotomy, at the time of delivery, but he now offers the Mark II as elective surgery. According to Burt, some 4000 women have had the surgery. Burt says that many of these operations were done experimentally during other surgical procedures without the women's knowledge.

Love surgery has not been well received in medical circles, and Burt says that he has become an outcast. According to one report, he has no academic affiliation and is not board-certified. His papers are turned down by respectable medical journals, and he is denied the opportunity to speak at medical meetings. Such was the fate of other pelvic surgeons before their ideas caught on. But even if Burt continues to be boycotted by colleagues, it should be noted that this form of censure only serves to isolate him from medical colleagues and to make his actions less, not more, visible. It does not prevent him from performing the surgery, as, indeed, he continues to do. See James C. Burt and Joan Burt, *Surgery of Love* (New York: Carlton Press, 1975).

92. "Transactions of the Women's Hospital Society," *American Journal of Obstetrics and Gynecology,* 43 (1901), 721.
93. Barker-Benfield, *Horrors,* pp. 120–121.
94. G. J. Barker-Benfield, "A Historical Perspective on Women's Health Care — Female Circumcision," *Women and Health,* 1 (1976), 13–20.
95. Engelmann, "American Girl," pp. 755–756.
96. William Mengert, *History of the American College of Obstetricians and Gynecologists, 1950–1970* (Chicago: American College of Obstetricians and Gynecologists, 1971).
97. J. E. Tyson, "The Attractiveness of Obstetrics and Gynecology as

a Professional Career," *American Journal of Obstetrics and Gynecology,* 117 (1973), 131.
98. Ibid., pp. 131–132.
99. James S. Krieger, "Of Fish and Fisherman," *American Journal of Obstetrics and Gynecology,* 116 (1973), 155–156.
100. Tyson, "The Attractiveness," p. 132.
101. Michael Newton and Frederick Zuspan, "A 1969 Profile of Residents in Obstetrics and Gynecology," *Obstetrics and Gynecology,* 38 (1971), 164.
102. Gordon Douglas, "The New Generation," *American Journal of Obstetrics and Gynecology,* 107 (1970), 151.
103. Seth Goldsmith, John Johnson, and Monroe Lerner, "Obstetricians' Attitudes Toward Nurse-Midwives," *American Journal of Obstetrics and Gynecology,* 111 (1971), 111–118.
104. William Keettel, "One Man's Opinion: Presidential Address," *American Journal of Obstetrics and Gynecology,* 115 (1973), 594.
105. Barbara Platte, "Board Sets Exams in First Three Ob. Gyn. 'Superspecialties,'" *Ob. Gyn. News* (March 15, 1974), 1.
106. David Burkons and J. Robert Willson, "Is the Obstetrician-Gynecologist a Specialist or Primary Physician to Women?" *American Journal of Obstetrics and Gynecology,* 121 (1975), 808–816; Howard C. Taylor, "Objectives and Principles in the Training of the Obstetrician-Gynecologist," *American Journal of Surgery,* 110 (1965), 35–42.

III

The Hospital Setting

A WOMAN OR MAN who becomes a fully trained physician in the United States today undergoes a number of years of education and clinical training. College is followed by medical school, where the first two years are spent studying the basic sciences in preparation for two years of clinical training. During the clinical years, medical students rehearse for future roles by performing simple tasks in a hospital, where, for the first time, they are exposed to people and to real medical problems.

Because twentieth-century medicine has become so specialized, most newly graduated physicians elect to concentrate in one area of medicine or surgery. After an optional year of internship, they enter a residency program. Residents, as these physician specialists-in-training are called, spend the next several years as the house staff in teaching hospitals, where they are responsible for treating people who, for various reasons, primarily economic ones, seek medical care through the clinics of teaching and public hospitals. Many residents, as we shall see, have no desire to serve this patient population but do so in order to acquire the skills of their chosen specialty. Elite Medical Center and Mass Hospital represent two different types of hospitals that train physicians and provide health care for the medically indigent.

Institution and Patients

Elite Medical Center is located on the periphery of a black, low-income area within a large industrial city. It is a large teaching- and research-oriented medical center that maintains an affiliation with a nearby university. Like most institutions, Elite claimed a special mission. Among its top priorities was the maintenance of an environment conducive to the intellectual growth of the professional staff.

The patient population at Elite was drawn from two sources: the private patients of the attending physician staff, and the institutional patients of the hospital's many clinics, for whom the resident house staff were responsible. The percentage of patients categorized as institutional was controlled through admissions procedures and policies. In obstetrics and gynecology, approximately 60 percent of the patients were private and consisted chiefly of white, middle- and upper-middle-class women; 40 percent were institutional and were largely black, working class, or poor. Both groups of patients shared the same facilities in the women's hospital within the Elite complex. The two groups' similarity ended with the facilities, because they received very different care.

• • •

Mass Hospital is located on the boundary between a major business and industrial district and a black low-income area in a big industrial city. Mass was reported to be one of the largest hospitals of its type in the United States. Though it had no primary university affiliation, clinical experience at Mass was prized by local medical students because of the hospital's reputation for treating a huge number of people with many different — sometimes rare — diseases. "You see everything at Mass" was a comment I frequently heard.

Mass did not provide facilities for private care. The patient population was entirely institutional and drawn primarily from the poor, black, and Spanish-speaking people of the city. Unlike other hospitals in the area, no one could be turned away from Mass Hospital. Consequently, the hospital received a large number of patients who were unwanted elsewhere. Mass estimated that each year approximately 53,000 patients were admitted to the hospital, more than 330,000 patients were seen in the emergency room, and 280,000 patients were treated in the hospital's outpatient clinics.

Like many public hospitals built early in the century, Mass was overcrowded and in need of repair. Though fresh paint added a bit of cheer, middle-class patients, accustomed to privacy and quiet, would find it a frightening and depressing place in which to be sick.

Most of the ob-gyn patients were assigned to huge open wards accommodating a minimum of twenty-eight beds. Heavy, opaque draw curtains provided privacy but were ineffective against noise. One large bathroom, which doubled as the patients' laundry room, was shared by all ward occupants. More important to women separated from their families for several weeks, the wards contained only two pay phones, equipped for outgoing but not incoming calls. These telephones were located in the hall some distance away from the beds, making them accessible only to ambulatory patients. Although the ob-gyn wards had been freshly painted and contained relatively new and bright furniture, it was the patients themselves who gave life to the wards and who made them a congenial place to be.

Privacy and solitude were at a premium, but friendship abounded. Patients literally took care of each other. An IV had little chance of running dry under the watchful eye of a ward mate. The women consoled, advised, and commiserated with each other over common problems, and they used each other's progress to gauge their own recoveries. In many ways, the women's wards resembled small communities where privacy was sacrificed but cooperation and neighborliness were gained.

It is impossible in this short treatment to do justice to the magnitude and complexity of Mass Hospital. It was an institution that contained a number of the new breed of young, radical physicians, specializing primarily in family practice, who were dedicated to improving the quality of health care for the urban poor. It was also an institution inevitably influenced by external political forces, constantly under fire from the community in which it was located, and divided by internal disorganization and dissension. Unlike Elite, the special mission at Mass placed greater emphasis on patient needs. In addition to providing medical education, Mass hoped to become an institution that could serve as a model for urban health care delivery.

Department and Staff

The Department of Obstetrics and Gynecology at Elite Medical Center was organized as one department under the central control of a Chair. In addition to its research and postresidency superspecialty training in gynecic endocrinology and infertility, the department had a full-time research staff engaged in a number of other continuing projects, and residents were expected and encouraged to participate.

Complementing the full-time research staff, there was the department's sizable attending staff of obstetrician-gynecologists. Besides utilizing Elite's facilities for their private patients, they taught and supervised medical students and residents. Each member of this staff was obligated to oversee the clinics and to spend some time on call, making himself available for consultations by the various resident services.

Because residents and attending physicians shared the same facilities, when problems arose an attending physician was frequently present and available for immediate consultation. This was especially common in labor and delivery, where residents and attendings spent many hours in the lounge, discussing cases while waiting for their patients to deliver.

Because there was physical proximity and considerable opportunity for informal contact between the two groups, social distance was somewhat reduced. Although most of the residents did not sense any closeness between themselves and the older attending staff — especially the Chair, who had the reputation of always "knowing what was going on" — the younger attending staff and residents were on a first-name basis and sometimes joined in social activities outside the hospital.

• • •

In contrast to Elite, the administration at Mass was often chaotic. The Department of Obstetrics and Gynecology was separated into two divisions under the central coordination of one department head. Each division was administered by a chief and one assistant. With the exception of the assistant chief of gynecology, whose function it was to administer the fellow program in gynecologic oncology (cancer of the female pelvis), all of the administrative and attending staff, including the Head, were in private practice at other hospitals. The amount of time they could spend at Mass was thus limited.

Based on my somewhat limited contact with the administration, it appeared that communication and cooperation between the two divisions of the department were minimal and that contact, when it did occur, was often characterized by enmity. Typical of departmental disorganization, the two divisions as well as the central administration were housed in different locations, further reducing the opportunity or inclination for communication. Toward the end of my field work, the department acquired a central location and moved into adjacent offices, which, it was hoped, would improve cooperation.

In a general sense, departmental problems were a reflection of the strain of functioning in an environment that encouraged competition for scarce resources. Because the two divisions were poorly integrated, internal problems tended to be seen in terms of one division or the other rather than of the department. If resident coverage in the labor room was inadequate, it was considered obstetrics' problem rather than the department's problem. The situation was complicated by a weak central administrator, who, for whatever reason, was frequently absent or unaware of specific internal problems. The schism and resulting discord affected both residents and patients, as will become clear.

In addition to the small part-time administrative staff, each division at Mass maintained a list of private attending physicians from the city whom residents could call for consultation on difficult cases and to assist at surgery. But unlike the arrangement at Elite, there was little incentive for attendings to spend much time at Mass since their private patients were treated elsewhere. In obstetrics one physician each night functioned as the night obstetrician and was on call for problems and emergencies on the labor row. All clinics were also supposed to be staffed with one attending physician. Although a few of these individuals could always be depended on, many were not reliable or simply did not take their obligation to Mass seriously. Residents frequently had difficulty locating an attending physician to supervise their surgery, which sometimes meant a case had to be canceled. The night obstetrician, according to residents — and this was borne out by my own observations — never slept in the hospital, as he was supposed to do. As a result, when emergencies occurred in labor and delivery there was almost always a delay in obtaining help.

Elite and Mass staff differed in several significant ways. Mass, because it was a public institution, had a large resident house staff and a small attending physician staff. Attendings used other hospital affiliations for their private patients. Because Elite was a semiprivate institution, the resident house staff and the attending staff utilized the same facilities to care for their patients. The result was the informal interaction between residents and attendings, noted above. And, what was important, there was a larger staff available to supervise and instruct residents in their activities at Elite.

The Residency Programs

Though a residency program is organized in good part to accommodate the residents' need for professional training, it must also perform a service for the hospital in which it is located. In a facility like Elite, the house staff assist the attending staff in the care and treatment of their private patients and also function as primary physicians for the hospital's institutional patient population. Thus, during his time in the program, the resident must cover a number of services, each of which has different value for him, depending on his personal training needs.

The residency period at Elite was four years long, with space for five residents at each year or level of training. The training year, commencing in July, was divided into five periods, or rotations, of approximately ten weeks each. They included the following services: clinic, labor and delivery, private gynecology, ward gynecology, and an elective.

During the ten weeks spent in the clinic, and much to their dislike, the residents had no opportunity to do deliveries or surgery. Clinic work consisted mainly of providing well care or preventive prenatal and gynecological care to a sizable number of institutional patients.

The rotation spent in the labor and delivery rooms consisted of twelve-hour daily shifts in which residents assisted attendings with their private patients and provided the primary source of care for institutional patients. Responsibilities included monitoring normal and high-risk labors, inducing labor, conducting deliveries, doing cesarean sections, and performing tubal ligations on postpartum women. The labor and delivery rooms served as a triage station for obstetrical patients, and residents provided emergency care and screened for false labor and pre-

TABLE 1

Service Rotations by Year of Training:
Elite Medical Center

First Year		*Second Year*	
Two rotations	— Labor and Delivery	Two rotations	— Labor and Delivery
One rotation	— Clinic	One rotation	— Private Gynecology
One rotation	— Private Gynecology	One rotation	— Ward Gynecology
One rotation	— Elective	One rotation	— Clinic

Third Year		*Fourth Year*	
One rotation	— Labor and Delivery (chief)	One rotation	— Obstetrics
One rotation	— Private Gynecology (chief)	Two rotations	— Ward Gynecology (one as chief)
One rotation	— Clinic (chief)	Two rotations	— Electives
Two rotations	— Electives		

eclampsia, a toxemia characterized by high blood pressure. Residents also performed circumcisions[1] and were responsible for the care of postnatal women on the wards.

Gynecology was divided into two services, private and ward. On private gynecology, the residents' main responsibility was to assist the attendings with their patients. This involved doing a certain amount of work that residents regarded as "undesirable," such as obtaining medical histories, doing physicals, making daily rounds, dictating surgical records, and the like. The reward, however, was being allowed to assist at or to do the attendings' surgery. In theory, while on the private service, the resident learned basic operative skills under the tutelage of experienced surgeons. On the ward service, residents had full responsibility for institutional patients. Work included diagnosis, surgery, and preoperative and postoperative care.

During the elective rotation, residents had the option of joining other medical or surgical departments within Elite for additional specialized training. The time could also be used to participate in departmental research or to engage in intensive work in gynecologic endocrinology and infertility. Most residents took advantage of the last option at least once during the four years, though some residents indicated that they often used the elective period as time off. Although they sometimes didn't comply, all residents were also expected to attend a daily lecture and weekly grand rounds, take part in a monthly residents' meeting and departmental dinner-business meeting, and spend several nights a month on call in the emergency room and assisting with obstetric or gynecologic problems that occurred elsewhere in the hospital.

During the total training period, a resident spent half of each year in obstetrics and half divided between ward and private gynecology. Consequently, ward and private services always contained junior residents and senior residents, with the most senior person acting as supervisor or chief resident of the service.

The structure and composition of ward and private gynecology services was important to residents; they significantly af-

TABLE 2

Services by Number of Residents at Each Level of Training: Elite Medical Center

Labor and Delivery	*Clinic*
Two first-year residents	One first-year resident
Two second-year residents	One second-year resident
One third-year resident (chief)	One third-year resident (chief)
Private Gynecology	***Ward Gynecology***
One first-year resident	One second-year resident
One second-year resident	Two fourth-year residents (rotating chief)
One third-year resident (chief)	

TABLE 3

Service Rotations by Year of Training after Change: Elite Medical Center

First Year	*Second Year*
Two rotations — Labor and Delivery	Two rotations — Labor and Delivery
One rotation — Private Gynecology	One rotation — Ward Gynecology
One rotation — Clinic	One rotation — Clinic
One rotation — Elective	
Third Year	***Fourth Year***
Two rotations — Private Gynecology (one as chief)	Two rotations — Ward Gynecology (one as chief)
One rotation — Labor and Delivery (chief)	Two rotations — Elective
One rotation — Clinic (chief)	One rotation — Obstetrics
One rotation — Elective	

TABLE 4

Services by Number of Residents at Each Level of Training after Change: Elite Medical Center

Labor and Delivery	*Clinic*
Two first-year residents	One first-year resident
Two second-year residents	One second-year resident
One third-year resident (chief)	One third-year resident
Private Gynecology	***Ward Gynecology***
One first-year resident	One second-year resident
Two third-year residents (rotating chief)	Two fourth-year residents (rotating chief)

fected the residents' ability to acquire certain types of experience during training. From a resident's perspective, the year in which a service was taken, whom one worked with on a service, the number of others on a service and their level of training, the sequence of rotations during the year as well as the time of year in which they were taken[2] — all were significantly related to the quality of the resident's individual training experience.

Slots in a residency program are not always filled. Though it happens infrequently, residents change programs or occasionally drop out, leaving an opening difficult to fill. Such was the case at Elite when a first-year resident decided to change programs at the end of the year, thus creating a vacancy in the second year. When it was announced that the vacancy was not going to be filled, a major dispute arose among residents about how the necessary basic changes in the residency program should be accomplished.

The controversy, which lasted for several weeks, centered on the fact that, because of the departing resident, there would be four rather than five residents in the second year, so the number of rotations for that year had to be reduced from five to four. The residents had to eliminate one of the two rotations in gynecology, either private or ward. Second-year residents were divided in their opinion about the relative training value of the two services; that is, which service enabled them to do the greatest amount of surgery. In the past, residents believed that the ward service provided a better opportunity to see medical problems and do surgery than did the private service. However, recent experience seemed to indicate that the attendings on the private service were allowing second-year residents to do more surgery than some chief residents on the ward service. The resolution of the dispute was further complicated because of the effect it would have on each of the other years.

If the ward gynecology rotation was eliminated during the second year, a replacement for the missing member of the service would have to come from either the first year or the third year, and this resident, along with the two fourth-year residents, would then constitute the ward service. Fourth-year residents argued that first-year residents were too inexperienced to provide the help necessary to run the ward service. Third-year residents reasoned that, with two fourth-year residents on the ward service claiming rank, they would be reduced to performing the most routine tasks.

If the private gynecology rotation was eliminated during the second year, third-year residents would have to substitute a second private gynecology rotation for one elective period in order to restore the private service to a full complement of residents. The objection to this solution came from residents who had had unsatisfactory experiences in private gynecology and were unwilling to spend a large segment of their third year on that service.

The issue was finally resolved, not to the satisfaction of all, by eliminating the private gynecology service from the second-year rotation. However, the intensity of the argument over these changes begins to illustrate the amount of negotiating that took place between residents as each vied for the opportunity to increase his personal share of surgical experience.

• • •

The residency program at Mass was as disorganized as the department in which it was located. Part of the problem was that the department was in the process of instituting changes in the organization of the program, and the result was often chaotic.

When I began my observations at Mass, the residency was a three-and-a-half-year program, not including a mandatory one-year internship. Unlike the majority of training hospitals, which have one starting date, July 1, at Mass four residents were admitted to the program twice a year, on January 1 and July 1. Thus, there was space for twenty-four residents in the program. That is, the entire first eighteen months were spent in obstetrics, with no exposure to gynecology; the entire second eighteen months were spent in gynecology, with no exposure to obstetrics. So it wasn't until the latter part of the second year, when residents were introduced to gynecology, that it was possible for them to begin to integrate the two fields. This type of organization also created a situation in which everyone on a service was at a similar stage of training, with no one possessing enough advanced experience to perform the role of teacher and supervisor for the service.

During the period on the obstetrical service, Mass residents spent time in three locations: the labor row, the prenatal clinic, and the ward for complicated obstetrics. New residents divided their time between the prenatal clinic and the labor row, where duties included supervising medical students, interns, and nurse-midwives; delivery of women who did not require surgery; monitoring of nonsurgical prenatal and postnatal women; and performing circumcisions. After nine to twelve months in the clinic and labor row, residents rotated to the ward for complicated obstetrics, where they were responsible for women who needed special care because they had, for example, diabetes or high blood pressure. These residents also performed all obstetrical surgery, including cesarean sections, operations for ectopic pregnancy, and tubal ligations on postpartum women.

During the second half of the second year, residents transferred to the gynecology service. During the eighteen months allocated to gynecology, residents also spent six weeks in the Department of Pathology, where they received training in diagnosis of diseased tissue, and six weeks in the emergency room. At Mass the emergency room was used not only for emergencies but as the main admissions area of the hospital as well. It operated at full capacity day and night, and each department was responsible for staffing the area with residents twenty-four hours a day. In obstetrics and gynecology, residents performed this service during their second year.

The gynecology division consisted of four services. Three handled similar types of problems. Different attending physicians were supposed to be assigned to each service, but in fact the number of attendings active at Mass was so small that all of the services tended to rely on the same individuals. Ideally, each service was supposed to have three residents — the number necessary to perform most surgery — each resident with a six-month difference in the length of training. These residents saw all of the patients in the gynecology clinics, cared for women with gynecological problems on other wards, and in addition were responsible for all the testing, diagnosis, surgery, management, and postoperative care of patients on their own service.

The fourth service was gynecologic oncology, and it consisted of a full-time attending, a fellow who had completed residency and was training as a specialist in oncology, a resident, and an intern. The experience an intern and resident received on this service was atypical: the teaching and supervision were excellent.

During the final six months of training, each resident rotated as chief through the labor row, complicated obstetrics, and gynecology. The responsibilities and duties of the chief, however, were never clearly defined, and each chief tended to interpret the role according to personal preference.

During the time spent in the gynecology division, residents had a number of additional duties. They were required to spend several weekends and evenings on call. Also, they were allowed to work in the evening family planning and abortion and counseling clinics, as well as to perform first-trimester abortions. Residents received additional pay for performing these services.

A variety of activities was planned for the residents and held more or less regularly. Friday was designated academic day, and no surgery was scheduled. Residents were expected to attend grand rounds, ward rounds, a basic science lecture, and a journal club meeting. The remainder of the week's activities included several topical lectures. Once a month an evening dinner-and-business meeting was scheduled.

At Mass, as at Elite, these activities were, in general, poorly attended by residents, especially those in the obstetrical division, largely because the activities were relevant to gynecology and were planned by that division.

This was the structure of the program when I began my observations at Mass. Shortly afterward, some changes began to occur. It was decided that the program would be reduced from three and a half years to three years and that new residents would be admitted in July only. The feeling was that better residents could be obtained in July, the traditional beginning of the medical year, and that residents who came in January were leftovers, who, for some reason, had been unable to find placements in July. That year, then, in January four residents completed the program and left Mass but were not replaced. Because the four new residents would have been assigned to obstetrics, that division suffered a serious staffing shortage. Gynecology, however, was also experiencing staffing problems, because a number of residents had been scheduled for their annual month vacation during the spring. During this period, conflict between the two divisions was apparent, as each attempted to work out its own staffing problems. For example, at one point the chief of gynecology was heard shouting at the chief of obstetrics that "if he really cared about patients, he would care about all of them, gynecology patients as well." (Field Notes, Mass.)

Mass residents also suffered under the strain of inadequate staffing, as these angry comments from a frustrated labor row resident indicate:

> I arrived on the labor row Sunday afternoon and met Dr. F., who was obviously in a bad mood. He was angry about the scheduling and remarked, "It should be very easy to make up schedules but they don't seem to be able to do it here. They let everyone take a vacation at the same time."
>
> He also said some residents were off to study for the Flex Exam. He was alone on the labor row, and they wanted to take his only intern to work in gynecology today because Dr. A., who was on call in the emergency room, was too busy to cover the wards. He said, "It's terrible how they run this place. Last week we were so short that they just arbitrarily promoted an intern to resident status so that he could write medication orders. We have to have two residents on the labor row at all times, and if we're short, they just promote an intern for a couple of days!" (Field Notes, Mass.)

On July 1, the situation at Mass became worse. Along with the decision to shorten the program to three years, it had been decided to make other changes in the program. Realizing the advantage to be gained from an integrated training in obstetrics and gynecology throughout the residency, the administration changed the program so that during each year residents would divide their time equally between obstetrics and gynecology.

As with the previous changes, obstetrics was somewhat more affected because half the incoming residents who would have started in obstetrics were now scheduled in gynecology. Advanced residents were also affected by the changes; after spending the allocated eighteen months in obstetrics, they were being asked to return to obstetrics. This would, and for some did, reduce their overall experience in gynecology to a seriously low level. Aware of the problem, the chief of gynecology told the residents:

> I am asking the third-year people to help me get this new program initiated. There will be lots of people in gynecology. They will be tripping over each other, but obstetrics is going to be short. The department has some responsibility to the patients in obstetrics, so I'm going to have to ask you to cooperate even though you aren't going to get exactly what you want. The attendings will have to cooperate and stretch the material available [that is, patients], because the people new to gynecology, who have so much obstetrical experience, will have to go back to obstetrics. We'll have to see to it that they get better than their share of cases. (Field Notes, Mass.)

Simply stated, the dilemma was that the patients needed residents in obstetrics but the residents needed experience in gynecology. Compromises were made between the divisions and schedules were changed, sometimes daily, in an effort to work out difficulties. This period was fraught with confusion for everyone concerned, including me. Not only did I have difficulty knowing where residents were supposed to be; they had the same difficulty. A labor row resident would report for duty on time, only to find the schedules had been changed and he wasn't due until eight hours later.

In spite of the administration's efforts to do the best for

patients and residents, given the new schedules, everyone involved in the change lost something. Obstetrics continued to be understaffed. The residents scheduled there were new and were required to work incredibly long hours. On the first couple of schedules, residents were expected to work twelve hours a day, with only one day off every other week, in what was considered to be one of the busiest labor rooms in the city. The complicated obstetrics ward was reduced to two residents responsible for all obstetrical complications and surgery, and they were scheduled to be on duty twenty-four hours a day, every other day. The situation prompted one resident to comment, "It is a complete mess and will be for a year." I responded that the moral was not to have your baby at Mass this year. He answered, "Just this year? Well, for sure not this summer."

At first, residents were not returned to obstetrics, but in time the labor room became so understaffed that something had to be done. The residents who were caught in this situation were forced to relinquish an important part of their time in gynecology. Of course, patient care at Mass during this period was affected, too.

Before the changes introduced at Mass, which occurred late in my field work, there were important differences in the structure of the two programs. At Mass, where the first eighteen months were spent in obstetrics and the second eighteen months in gynecology, services had residents at similar levels of training and skill, thus reducing the potential for peer supervision and teaching. At Elite, where obstetrics and gynecology were integrated over the four-year training period, services were hierarchical and had residents at various levels of training. Because of the dissimilarity in the two programs, as well as institutional and departmental differences, Elite and Mass provided an interesting contrast on which to base an analysis of surgical training and patient care.

The Residents

The profession of obstetrics and gynecology, and medicine in general, is overwhelmingly dominated by men. It is not surprising that the majority, 76 percent, of residents at Elite and Mass were males. At Elite, out of 23[3] residents, 5 were female, and at Mass 6 of the 24 residents were female.

Elite, because of its prestigious position, attracted a larger number of American medical school graduates than did Mass. Ten of the twenty-three Elite residents were foreign-born and -educated, two were black, and one was Puerto Rican, in contrast to Mass, where nineteen of twenty-four were foreign and 5 were black. All of the females in both programs, except one black woman, were foreign.

Most of the foreign residents came to the United States because they expected the medical training here to be better than in their own countries. As one resident put it, "I made a sacrifice by giving up all my friends. I lived in luxury there. I had no financial problems. I was really living happy there and I came here to a new environment, not hostile, to a different world, and I sort of gave up all my small warm things that I used to have just for the sake of good medicine." (Interview, Elite.)

As might be expected, Elite residents were more likely to come from professional families; 56 percent of those interviewed did, but only 36 percent of the Mass residents interviewed came from professional backgrounds. Twenty-one percent of Mass residents and only 11 percent of Elite residents had working-class backgrounds. These distinctions are important, because wide class differences between physician and patient affect communication and, in turn, treatment.

The average age of the residents was twenty-nine; all but a few were married; and most of the male residents had children. At Mass, two of the female residents were pregnant. One was just beginning to wear maternity clothes when I concluded my research; the other had her baby while I was still there. Wishing to prove that pregnancy needn't hinder a physician, this second woman resident carried a full work load up to the day she went into labor, and refused all offers of help from her colleagues. She commented to me,

> "They think you can't do the job other doctors do. But I didn't have any problems. I kept working up till the last

> moment so they can't say anything. Doing a vaginal hysterectomy in the last months is very difficult because the table is just right there and there isn't enough room. But I did abdominal hysterectomies. There was no problem because you can raise the table or stand on a stool." (Interview, Mass.)

"The Happy Specialty"

During the process of this research I frequently have been asked why men choose to become obstetrician-gynecologists. Do "gynecologists love women collectively probably more than most men do," as the anonymous author of *Confessions of a Gynecologist*[4] stated? Or is the more skeptical view, that they hate women, true? I talked to the residents about their career choice and about women as patients. They may not represent the whole profession, but their responses give insight in the matter.

Medical students consider a number of factors when deciding on which specialty to enter. The nature of the work, the intellectual content of the specialty, the length of residency, the type of patient encountered, individual psychological compatibility with the work, income, and hours — all are considered.

Residents consistently mentioned the same aspects of an obstetrician-gynecologist's work as what attracted them to the field. They called obstetrics and gynecology the "happy specialty" because the majority of problems are curable and because the residents believed their patients were grateful.

> I think you get a lot of satisfaction from this field because the patients come to see you and they always go out happy. In medicine you have patients lying there for ages and you can't do anything about it. Ob is a happy field and I like it. (Interview, Mass.)

In general, residents didn't begin medical school committed to a career in obstetrics and gynecology. Rather, they arrived at the decision through a process of elimination as they progressed through the clinical years, gaining exposure in each specialty.

> I took surgery . . . and decided I didn't want to do surgery exclusively. I didn't want all that blood and guts. I didn't want to walk around dripping blood all the time, though actually ob is more surgery than I thought . . . I couldn't be a pediatrician. I started to be a psychiatrist but then I thought that was a waste. I would have wasted all that time taking physiology, etc.; I could just have gotten a Ph.D. in psychology.
>
> I got into ob through elimination of what I didn't want. Ob was my last rotation and I didn't want peds, didn't want general surgery, and psychiatry . . . So I got to ob by default and I said I just really hope I like it, and I did. Now maybe that was because I said that I had to like it but anyway that's how I got into it. (Interview, Mass.)

A few residents were originally attracted to surgery and chose obstetrics and gynecology because it covered a limited anatomical region of one sex and was relatively simpler to master than general surgery. As one resident said, "It takes five to six years to be a general surgeon, and then you have to spend three or four more years getting a subspecialty. I wanted something that, after a period of time, I would know all of, not like general surgery where you never know it all." (Interview, Mass.)

The majority of residents, however, were originally attracted to obstetrics. As medical students, they found delivering babies fun; childbirth also provided an element of drama that appealed to them. Observations of medical students during their first delivery generally confirm this.

> J., a new medical student on the service, had just done his first delivery and was very excited. He kept talking about how cute the baby was. In fact he sounded like a proud father. He told me that this baby was going to know what he wanted and get it. To prove it he said his head

> had been born while they were still scrubbing; he hadn't even waited for them. (Field Notes, Elite.)

Within medicine, obstetrician-gynecologists are said to have a "cure complex." That is, residents derived satisfaction from surgical intervention and were frustrated by less aggressive medical treatment. The potential for successful surgical intervention was another factor that attracted residents to the field.

> I think that ob-gyn is a very happy field in medicine, especially obstetrics. Of course there are sad moments, but they are rare in comparison to other specialties. It is very rewarding and I think that they [doctors] are looking for very immediate reward. A doctor that is in medicine, for example, checking all those pulmonary edemas, etc., he knows that he is not going to cure. He knows that sooner or later this man is going to come back . . .
>
> But I don't know, for me at least, I don't feel that he is really curing the people, and in obstetrics you have a woman coming into the labor room, she is in pain, you try to give her a good time in the labor room, and she delivers and she is happy and the baby is fine, the mother is fine and they go home, and you did something. The same in gyn. I'm not talking about oncology, but the fibroids and the routine things you see in gyn, the enlarged uterus, the anatomical things we correct — the patient is not really suffering too much with this. After the hysterectomy you feel you have really corrected it. (Interview, Elite.)

"Ego Trip"

Because, in contrast to the poor, middle-class women enjoy relatively better general health, nutrition, and medical care, their deliveries are usually without medical complications, and the obstetrician, though he may have contributed little, appears successful. For many residents, this was an "ego trip."

> I think the most important thing is it's relatively pleasant, it's a little bit of an ego trip, obstetrics is. Generally you know the deck is stacked in your favor, you're going to come out with a good outcome no matter what. In spite of that, the patient thinks you're wonderful and great. So it's an ego trip. (Interview, Elite.)

If obstetrics bolsters the practitioner's ego, infertility work is an even greater ego trip.[5] For one thing, married women seeking assistance to become pregnant exhibit traditional sex-role behavior. Unmarried women, on the other hand, were usually refused referral to the infertility clinic. Expertise in reproductive endocrinology also provides the practitioner with the skill to control women's reproductive potential. The sexual overtones were unmistakable, and residents frequently bragged excitedly about "getting their patients pregnant." A departing resident who planned a career in reproductive endocrinology and infertility remarked:

> I think it's a big kick to see a patient for the first time, make the appropriate diagnosis, institute the appropriate therapy, and end up with a healthy baby. Once in a while it might be a kick to deliver that patient too, but it is more of a kick just to get her pregnant. And again it's an ego trip because the girls in our office who get pregnant think that we are great . . . The transference between patients and even routine obstetrics is an interesting thing to study and it certainly goes on. Often I have seen the transference to be of such an incredible degree that the husband ends up, at least in the wife's eyes, as playing a very insignificant role. Almost as if the doctor was in bed with her on that fateful night rather than the husband. (Interview, Elite.)

Emphasis on Life — Avoidance of Death

The obverse of the emphasis placed by residents on youth, fertility, and life is their strong negative attitude toward those aspects of medicine which necessitated dealing with terminal illness and death. A decided advantage of obstetrics and gynecology is that not only can the male practitioner dissociate his own mortality from the pathology he sees, but he also has to confront death only infrequently in the normal process of his work.

> To tell you the truth it was more a decision by exclusion. I really didn't like most of the other specialties . . . At least in ob you are dealing with young people who by and large have a pretty good outcome. Most of them are satisfied with the outcome. You aren't dealing most of the time with any serious life-threatening condition where you have people dying all the time. You may lose one or two now and then on a gyn service but rarely on an ob service. (Interview, Elite.)
>
> It's a happy service, basically happy. Things can be bad, ladies screaming. Cesarean sections can be bad but basically when it's all over, they still have that smile on their face . . . In surgery, they are operating on really old people and on medicine you have these really brittle diabetics and cardiacs and you know as soon as they get better and go home, they will be back, and that's depressing. There has only been one death that I have been involved in since I came here. (Interview, Mass.)

Death, in a sense, is viewed as antithetical to the "life thrust" of obstetrics and gynecology. It has been suggested that because of this, and because of the infrequency with which death is confronted, death may pose special problems for obstetrician-gynecologists.[6]

The residents' attitudes toward abortion also appeared to be related to the emphasis on life in obstetrics and gynecology. Most residents, although they didn't want to be known as "abortion doctors," expected to do first-trimester abortions in private practice, primarily for personal economic reasons. First trimester abortion was acceptable as long as women were not suspected of using it as a form of birth control. Second-trimester abortion, however, was viewed in a substantially different light.

> I don't like doing abortions but I probably will because of the economics of it . . . Midtrimester is very distasteful to me. I really don't get a kick out of doing them, I don't know too many guys who enjoy doing them. (Interview, Elite.)

> I cannot see myself fighting on the one hand to save a baby and on the other hand expediting its expulsion. I think if a woman has gone by the first trimester and is thinking of an abortion, she should place [the baby] up for adoption. There are a lot of people that can't have children. (Interview, Mass.)

> I have no strong feelings against first-trimester abortions. They don't disturb me at all. Midtrimester abortions I find esthetically unpleasant. I don't think it is from a religious perspective necessarily; I just find them unpleasant. I guess it is difficult for me to excuse a woman for waiting until she is fourteen or sixteen weeks pregnant to make up her mind she doesn't want it, but aside from that it just goes against everything we have been training for. (Interview, Elite.)

Residents seemed to be unable to reconcile their obstetrical objective, the delivery of a viable infant, with the performance of second-trimester abortions, and many disapproved of women who sought them. Self-determination for women is not likely to become a major goal of the specialty soon. Even those residents who indicated that women should be able to obtain abortions also said they would not personally perform them unless forced by economic necessity. Given this evidence, it is reasonable to question obstetricians' monopoly on abortion and to ask whether women would not be better served by a group psychologically better prepared for the work.

Residents were also attracted by the relative youth of their clientele. Young women are not only productive but reproductive, and thus possess social worth, a highly valued characteristic in patients. As one resident commented, "I don't know, it's just a good field. It's associated with life and young people and for the most part happy things, and that's why I like it." (Interview, Elite.)

Residents believed that practitioners of the happy specialty were basically different from other surgeons. They were "jollier," more conservative about "cutting," and less constrained by matters of professional status and hierarchy. One resident, whose father was a general surgeon, explained:

> They are more relaxed, the gyn people. As a whole, if you have to classify the two, they are much more relaxed, not as aggressive. A surgeon is always ready to cut, period, at least the ones I know, and they are also very hierarchical in terms of: I am the surgeon and you are the second and you are the first and you do what you are told and shut up. Whereas in gyn it seems to be a lot more relaxed and the status is more blurred. There isn't as much of a hierarchy thing as there is a pitch-together type of thing. (Interview, Mass.)

Control over Women

It has been suggested that men choose to become obstetrician-gynecologists because of an underlying ambivalence or hostility toward women and a desire to control a group less powerful than themselves. There is evidence to suggest that power and control are important to the obstetrician-gynecologist. In fact, several residents suggested that rather than interview them, I should administer personality tests to them; they believed that as a group they would score relatively high on manipulative or Machiavellian items. Instead, I talked to them about their preference in patients and about the types of attitudes they thought women should have.

Every resident indicated a preference for educated rather than uneducated women. However, "educated," as the residents used it, did not mean women who possessed the power of reasoning and judgment or the ability to make knowledgeable decisions. Rather, the term as they used it described middle-class women with middle-class values; that is, those who placed a high premium on good health and who had been taught to respect and submit to the authority of experts. Poor people, the residents believed, lacked middle-class values, were casual about health matters, failed to respond to medical authority, and did not exhibit appropriate deference to physicians. In short, the residents preferred "happy," obedient, respectful, and thankful patients.

> I like an educated woman. I don't like women that think they know more than the doctor and who complain about things that they shouldn't be complaining about. (Interview, Elite.)

> I think the main thing is that the patient understands what I say, listens to what I say, does what I say, believes what I say. (Interview, Elite.)

> I don't care for the patient that gives you a fight every time you try to give them a drug. I don't care for the patient that disagrees with me. And I don't care for the patient that wants me to cure her but won't do anything to help. (Interview, Elite.)

> Somebody that is interested and cares, will listen to the things that you say, and calmly do what you tell them. (Interview, Elite.)

Residents did express a strong desire to control their patients, but whether this characteristic sets them apart from other types of physicians is debatable. Obstetrician-gynecologists may differ from other physicians in one respect, however. There is evidence that residents believed their prospective patients, middle-class women, were more malleable and submissive to authority than men. Given the combination of class, sex, and the authority invested in the doctor, male obstetrician-gynecologists are able to experience a sense of power and control over their female clients.

> I think we have less problems because our patients are women. I think women are easier to handle than men, easier to talk to in a way. They listen more; they may even believe you. I think it is easier to treat them. (Interview, Mass.)
>
> I enjoy taking care of those patients because they are young patients and it is nice to deal with them. They are young, they don't give you a hard time, they listen to you. And you treat them and they get pregnant; it's a really nice thing. They are so thankful to you. (Interview, Mass.)

But many women are neither complacent about nor pleased with their obstetrical and gynecological care. They are insulted by paternalistic physicians who expect them to act like happy, obedient children. The loss of reproductive organs is more likely to be a cause for mourning than rejoicing, and birth is sometimes experienced as a depressing rather than a joyous event. From this perspective, the happy specialty is a contradiction in terms created by male practitioners who, because they cannot experience the problems they treat, tend to trivialize or misinterpret the significance these problems hold for women.

Would Women Be Better Obstetrician-Gynecologists Than Men?

Women outnumber men in the total health care labor force, but they occupy the lower-paid, less prestigious positions in the medical hierarchy, such as nurse, physical or occupational therapist, social worker, and service worker. The power continues to be concentrated in the hands of white, upper-middle-class males. How health care would change if women rather than men held positions of power is open to debate.

Some argue that class loyalty is stronger than sex loyalty.[7] Consequently, increasing the number of women in medical school would not improve the position of all women in health care because, according to this argument, female physicians are closer to, and more supportive of, male physicians than of their working-class sisters. Advocates of this position argue that people with working-class backgrounds must be recruited into the medical profession and positions of power.

The effect of this strategy, unless it is accompanied by a change in our health care system, isn't clear. For one thing, medical school exerts a strong influence with lasting effects; there is pressure on everyone to engage in the same behavior in order to "make it." This is not meant to imply that women have not brought or cannot bring about change, but it does suggest that medical socialization favors the status quo. In spite of this, my data, though based on a small number of women (eleven), indicate that female residents were different from their male colleagues in at least one significant way.

None of the women at Elite or Mass would be considered a feminist in terms of the ideology and goals of the women's movement in America. In the societies from which most of the female residents came, female physicians were more numerous than in the United States and were not considered sex-role deviants. Because of cultural taboos, obstetrics and gynecology was considered to be most appropriately a woman's specialty. The female residents came from backgrounds that were very different from their patients', but because they had personally experienced many of the same problems, they were more empathic than the males. They were also more likely to take certain symptoms seriously and less likely to conclude that illnesses were psychogenic.

British physicians K. Jeanne Lennane and R. John Lennane[8] argue that several conditions specific to women, including dysmenorrhea (menstrual pain or cramps), nausea during pregnancy, and pain in labor, are commonly considered to be caused or aggravated by psychogenic factors, although scientific evidence clearly implicates organic factors.

Menstrual pain, for example, is a well-defined clinical entity dependent, in part, on ovulation. When ovulation is suppressed, as it is with the use of oral contraceptives, menstrual pain is either absent or significantly decreased. The Lennanes state that despite the fact that the association between dysmenorrhea and ovulation has been known for over thirty years, gynecology textbooks still emphasize a psychosomatic explanation. Some texts state that "the pain is always secondary to an emotional problem"; others assert that women who have menstrual pain are high-strung, nervous or neurotic, or are ambivalent about their role as wives or mothers.

In her book on menstruation and menopause, Paula Weideger[9] observes that even though menstrual pain is a monthly experience for very many women, relatively little research has been done on a cure.

In a related observation, Weideger discusses the menstrual taboo, a worldwide and persistent belief that connects impurity and danger with women's sexual processes. Pliny the Elder (A.D. 23–79) wrote that menstrual blood was a fatal poison that could destroy insects, cause fruit to fall from branches, and dull razors. Although attitudes are more enlightened today, myths about menstruation still exist. The continuing belief in psychosomatic causes suggests that in our times there remains something mysterious about woman's monthly bleeding.

Residents were encouraged to suspect that many "female complaints," including menstrual pain, were psychosomatic, but female residents were less likely than their male counterparts to accept these explanations, as the following remark indicates:

> Well if you have a patient with severe dysmenorrhea, this patient is really suffering every month. They [males] will tell her, take some aspirin. They will never know. You tell a doctor you are having headaches, you know hormonal headaches like premenstrual headaches, or when you are on birth control pills, with sudden withdrawal of hormones you can have bad headaches. They will never understand that.
>
> Dysmenorrhea — they just think the patient is having some cramps. They probably had some diarrhea in their life and they think this is the same. They just don't understand. From studying about dysmenorrhea they won't

> understand that the uterus is contracting and is giving pain to the woman in the same way that cervical dilation is painful in a woman. (Interview, Mass.)

The Lennanes make a similar point about the pain associated with childbirth. They assert that there is a widely held belief, largely because of natural childbirth theory, that this pain is also psychogenic in origin. Although it is known that strong visceral contractions against an obstruction are painful, the theory postulates that the pain is due to an increase in muscular tension caused by fear and that if the fear is removed, the pain will be, too. The Lennanes point out that it is remarkable to expect the prevention of an emotional response will remove the sensation itself. They observe that the theory seems to work in practice mainly by the woman's refusal to accept that pain is, in fact, present.

It is not my intention to argue the relative merits of natural childbirth, but there are a few points worth noting. At Elite, the majority of private patients had Lamaze deliveries. There are important benefits to be derived from Lamaze, not the least of which is the presence of a laboring woman's advocate in the labor and delivery rooms to provide support and ensure courteous treatment by the staff. If behavior can be taken as any indication of pain, a large number of these women, especially as they went through the second stage of labor, were having far from painless experiences. However, especially in the early stage of labor, they were usually more controlled and screamed less than institutional patients who had not been taught Lamaze techniques.

Birth room personnel responded negatively toward laboring women who screamed. From the residents' point of view, the ideal delivery was one in which the woman was "nicely controlled." However, as the Lennanes make clear, controlling one's response to pain does not mean the pain is not there. Residents, however, were often heard denying that what these women felt was pain. They told institutional patients that they were feeling "a little pressure and discomfort," and backed up this statement by comparing the difference in response to labor between Lamaze and non-Lamaze women. The residents' belief that pain was not real is important, because institutional patients who screamed during labor received harsh treatment.

When questioned about the amount of pain in childbirth, male residents invariably invoked psychological explanations:

> By their personality they can make the pain better or tolerable. There is a lot of psychology in this. When I put my hand there [on the abdomen] I feel exactly what is going on; I know if it is hurting. Everyone has experience with spastic pain whatever it is. If it is gastrointestinal or the problem in the army with diarrhea . . . afterward you experience this spastic pain. (Interview, Elite.)
>
> . . . The reaction to pain is psychological. The neuro input is real . . . We aren't seeing the neurons being stimulated, we are seeing how the patients react. In labor, the woman's attitude toward pain, her attitude toward childbearing, understanding of labor, self-control, these affect the subjective response to pain. I imagine it is less than a kidney stone but more than a sprained ankle. (Interview, Elite.)

In contrast, female residents who had themselves experienced childbirth talked about pain in a markedly different way. Because of their subjective understanding of the experience, they were more considerate, patient, and empathic toward women in labor.

> Men are unable to tolerate pain. Men would never be able to tolerate labor pain, they can't tolerate a toothache, so they will never be able to understand it. They don't go through it and they won't understand it. When I am at the bedside of a patient feeling her painful contraction, trying to give her some relief, I feel it much more than the men can. I am involved. The man can feel she has a pain;

> probably give her something. I will suffer with the patient; they won't, never, never. (Interview, Mass.)

Another female resident commented:

> I think that women would probably be better in ob especially if they have had babies because they understand what it is like. When I was here, several patients I had, screaming, yelling, and hollering, said, "I can't stand to have my legs up in these stirrups" and I said, "Yes I know" and she said, "No you don't" and I said, "Yes I do because I have had three!" She said, "You have had three babies?" and I said, "Sure" and she said, "OK I'll do whatever you say."
>
> So you can sympathize with them, you know how it feels and if you make them believe that you are trying to help because you understand how painful it is, then you can work with them and they will work with you . . . I think that a woman can sympathize more with childbirth than men; you know they have never experienced it. They do it [deliveries] every day but they never physically experienced it. (Interview, Elite.)

Female residents were observed to undergo attitudinal and behavioral changes once they themselves had experienced childbirth, as one female resident in commenting on a colleague makes clear:

> If the woman has delivered herself she knows what labor pains are, you know. They experience them and they are more gentle. Like one of the residents with us. I know what she was like before and she was totally different after she had her baby because she had experienced the labor pains herself. She was so rude to the patients before. When the patients on the labor row were in pain she would shout at them; she couldn't stand anybody shouting, you know. And after she had the baby, you could see

> the change. Now she has so much patience. (Interview, Mass.)

One resident who gave birth to her first child during residency spoke about her conversion experience:

> Well, reading it in books and experiencing it yourself is different. So when I experienced that it is really that painful, I thought, "Oh, my God, now I know what my patients are feeling" . . . To experience it yourself is different because you have that feeling, you know how painful it is. Because you really can't describe the pain, it is the kind of pain that is so painful. Oh, my God! (Interview, Mass.)

Interestingly, one male resident also spoke of a change in attitude after he had "experienced" his wife's delivery. In response to the question, "Can you describe labor pain?" he said:

> Yes, only because my wife had a baby. If she didn't have a baby, I probably couldn't describe it. Because when she was in labor, I swear to you, I felt every contraction she had, every single contraction.
>
> [Q. Why was it different with your wife?]
>
> Because I cared more for her than anybody else. If I have a patient that I don't know over here and she says, "Oh, it hurts," I don't feel anything but when my wife said it hurt, I really felt it . . . I was taught in medical school how pain is psychological. Then when I would see a girl in labor and she would be hollering, I would think it is all in her head, it's nothing. When my wife went through it — she isn't the kind of girl that says ouch very much — and when she said ouch, I said this isn't psychological, this is real pain. (Interview, Elite.)

Physicians traditionally have rejected the idea that personal experience is relevant to medical treatment. It isn't necessary, they argue, to have had cancer in order to operate successfully on a malignant tumor. But the capacity to care is also important, and it is not a quality that necessarily develops along with the skill to dispense medical remedies. Part of the purpose of this book is to demonstrate that while institutional patients were receiving medical treatment, they also suffered from an acute lack of caring. In the specific case of women's health problems, the female residents demonstrated that in spite of their medical training, they had a greater capacity for understanding than did their male colleagues. Male physicians will continue to be preferred by some, but if these eleven women are typical, as I suspect future research will confirm, then an increase in the number of women in the happy specialty would provide a welcome alternative.

Notes

1. Although obstetricians' responsibility for the newborn terminates at birth, they do perform circumcisions because pediatricians are not surgeons. Circumcision involves surgery without local anesthesia and is the most inhuman ritual I have ever observed. Physicians claim that the infant will forget, but even if they are right, the procedure is no less painful while it is going on.
2. There is less surgery scheduled during the summer and winter holiday seasons because patients are less willing to be confined in a hospital during these times. For a further discussion of the effect of scheduling on training experience, see Chapter VI.
3. This figure is larger than the number of openings in the program because my observations extended over the start of a new medical year and take into account five rather than four cohorts.
4. Anonymous, M.D., *Confessions of a Gynecologist* (New York: Doubleday, 1972).
5. Residents also described surgery as an "ego trip." Suddenly, in the middle of an operation one afternoon, it occurred to me that the ritual taking place in the surgical suite was very similar to the ritual I had observed many times as a child attending a Catholic mass. Obviously, men are the principal actors in both dramas. An important act in each is the ritual cleansing, which symbolizes purity and takes the form of the washing of the hands. Because surgeon and priest have been purified and touch only sterilized or consecrated objects, nurses must gown and assist the surgeon in

the same way that altar boys must robe and assist the priest. The manner in which a scrubbed surgeon holds his hands, up and parallel to his face, is similar to the way in which a consecrated priest holds his hands before handling the host. Patients are draped in a manner reminiscent of the ritual with the altar cloths. And medication and solutions are poured into sterile crucibles before use by the surgeon in the same way that wine, representing blood, is ritualized in the mass. The surgical scene is overlaid with seriousness until the organ or infant is removed, in the same way that the mass remains serious until after the offertory. And like the priest, the surgeon exits first, leaving his assistants to complete the less sacred tasks. In a sense, this imagery suggests that both surgeon and priest are the officiants at a sacrifice.

6. John Astrachan, "The Critically Ill Patient and the Gynecologist," *American Journal of Obstetrics and Gynecology* 116 (1973), 126.
7. Vicente Navarro, "Women in Health Care," *New England Journal of Medicine* 292 (1975), 398–402.
8. K. Jeanne Lennane and R. John Lennane, "Alleged Psychogenic Disorders in Women — A Possible Manifestation of Sexual Prejudice," *New England Journal of Medicine* 288 (1973), 288.
9. Paula Weideger, *Menstruation & Menopause: The Physiology and Psychology, the Myth and the Reality* (New York: Alfred Knopf, 1976).

IV

The Surgical Mentality

> If like all human beings, he [the gynecologist] is made in the image of the Almighty, and if he is kind, then his kindness and concern for his patient may provide her with a glimpse of God's image.
>
> — Russell C. Scott, M.D.[1]

Skills Emphasized in Training

Belita Cowan characterized physicians as "M.D.eities." The monopoly physicians have been able to maintain over medical knowledge has served to mystify the public about health and create the belief that medicine is too complicated for the average person to understand. Historically, the medical profession has been able to maintain autonomy or freedom from outside regulation on the basis of their claim to specialized knowledge.

Eliot Freidson[2] points out that it is often assumed that physicians have expertise in areas where they actually have no more knowledge than the rest of the public. He suggests that in order to evaluate the physician's claim to expertise, it is necessary to evaluate what he is trained to know and to do. These are especially pertinent questions, since a physician's authority derives, in good measure, from his status as an expert. Since obstetrician-gynecologists, because of their special training, are designated the official and legitimate experts on women, it is important for women to understand the limits of their expertise.

An analysis of what obstetrician-gynecologists are trained to do, as opposed to the actual content of their work, should shed light on such issues as unnecessary surgery. A look at what obstetrician-gynecologists are not trained to do should reveal the priorities and orientation of members of the profession.

What an Obstetrician-Gynecologist Is Trained to Do

Within specialties there are certain core skills considered prerequisites for certification as a practicing professional. They are part of almost every training program. In obstetrics and gynecology, in addition to surgical skill, they include knowledge of anatomy, physiology, pathology, and diseases related to fertility control, pregnancy, and the female reproductive tract and genital organs. Other skills are not acquired by everyone in the profession, but only by those who are trained in departments in which the superspecialty is represented. Finally, there are some skills that neither Elite nor Mass emphasized in training and that appear to be neglected in the profession generally.

> A good ob-gyn needs to have, first, good technical skills, good operative skills. He has to be fairly meticulous in his technique and dissection and he also has to know how to think on his feet and make the right judgment. And not only is it a matter of putting the clamps a certain way or the rote repetition of doing surgery but I think the good surgeons around here, and the type of surgeon that I want to be, is the kind that is well trained, knows a lot of different techniques, and knows when to use them and how to make decisions because a lot of good surgery is making the right decisions, judgment. (Interview, Elite.)

> Well, I think he has to be a good clinician first. That means he should keep up with medicine, not only the gyn part but all diseases that might affect women. It is also important to have some degree of surgical skill. He should be able to do the basic procedures. (Interview, Mass.)

When residents were asked to name the most important qualities needed by a good obstetrician-gynecologist they answered "medical judgment" and "surgical skill." Their highest priority was consistent with the historical and contemporary emphasis within the profession: surgical experience. Training developed in residents a sense of identity closely linked to the role of surgeon and thus taught them to achieve their primary work satisfaction from the act of operating.

> You open the belly, you know what you are doing, you take something out, and the patient gets better, and you know your diagnosis, and you have helped the patient. So I think that is the most satisfactory thing. That is the main thing. You know what you are doing, you take it out, and the patient gets better. (Interview, Mass.)

> I don't know, it is the same thing as in kindergarten when you took a little car apart . . . The thing with surgery is that you have something to show. You have a headache and I give you an aspirin and it goes away, fine. If you have postpartum bleeding and you need a hysterectomy and I take your uterus out and everything is fine, you can say, "look at that fine piece of surgery I did." (Interview, Mass.)

> Surgery is, well, to go and open someone up, take out an organ and close him up again and have him live; it tends to inflate your ego. (Interview, Mass.)

Another source of emphasis in residents' training came from the specific orientation of the faculty at Elite and Mass, each of which represented a different superspecialty within obstetrics and gynecology. Residents at Elite emerged from training with some specialized skill in gynecologic endocrinology and infertility. Mass residents lacked all but superficial knowledge of the most elemental principles in this specialty area, but they were exposed to and had performed radical surgery for uterine cancer because of the department's specialization in oncology. Elite residents were almost totally lacking in this type of operative skill.

The training program for obstetrician-gynecologists at Mass and Elite emphasized the types of skills needed to handle pathological conditions and acute situations. These skills were linked to a dependency on an array of medical hardware, such as fetal monitoring machinery. Residents learned to define medical practice in terms of this model, but one wonders whether the model accurately defines the average physician's daily office practice.

At Elite and Mass, in spite of their exposure to specialty skills, only a few residents expected to undergo the additional training required for ABOG certification as a superspecialist. At Elite, residents, though they thought they could use their infertility training in private practice, were also aware that relatively few women are in need of this service. At Mass, because of the complexity of extensive uterine cancer surgery, none of the residents, in spite of his training, felt skilled enough to perform this type of surgery without a fully trained oncologist at his side. In short, the large majority of residents expected to enter into a general group practice, where there would be little opportunity to practice the specialty skills acquired in training.

Despite the surgical and superspecialty emphasis of training for the profession, the average obstetrician-gynecologist is more likely to function as a general practitioner for his clients. A study published in 1975 found that of 1000 patients of fifty-one Michigan obstetrician-gynecologists, 44 percent had no primary care physician, and 86 percent saw only their obstetrician-gynecologist for regular periodic checkups. Forty-one percent reported that their obstetrician-gynecologist had treated them for a nongynecological condition or had decided that no treatment was necessary.[3]

In 1965 it was estimated that the annual work load of an average obstetrician-gynecologist consisted of 200 deliveries, 8 cesarean sections, 2000 antepartum and postpartum visits, 10 spontaneous abortions, 10 cases of infertility, 16 abdominal hysterectomies, 10 operations on the ovaries, 7 vaginal procedures, and an undetermined number of visits for minor gynecological complaints and regular pelvic examinations.[4] It is evident that in 1965 the average obstetrician-gynecologist was performing relatively few major surgical procedures.* This reflects the fact that women have more routine obstetrical and gynecological problems than they have conditions that require surgery.

What a Woman's Doctor Is Not Taught

Not only is the obstetrician-gynecologist trained in certain skills that are infrequently required in his work, but he is trained to derive his chief source of satisfaction from performing these skills. On the other hand, he is not trained in — nor does he learn to gain satisfaction from — other skills he will be called on to use in private practice. Here it is important to make a distinction between the typical practice of an obstetrician-gynecologist and the typical practice of a surgeon or superspecialist. The surgeon or superspecialist has relatively short-term relationships with patients and limited opportunity to engage in personal interaction with them. In contrast, the obstetrician-gynecologist, as a primary physician, has relatively long-term relationships with patients, many of whom come to expect certain expertise from their physicians.

Because the obstetrician-gynecologist is the "official" expert on the female reproductive tract and handles matters peripherally involved in sexuality, such as infertility and family planning, women have come to assume that their physicians possess expert knowledge, or some knowledge, of human, especially female, sexuality. And because the obstetrician-gynecologist tends to be consulted more frequently than other types of physicians, especially during a woman's reproductive years, he is often the one with whom she will discuss her emotional and sexual problems. It is important, then, to understand how un-

* It should be remembered that during the early sixties the birth rate was still high and the obstetrical business still lucrative. The result was that most of a physician's time was spent providing routine obstetrical and gynecological well care.

trained and unprepared many obstetrician-gynecologists are to handle these important problems.

Several years ago, Pauline Bart and I did an analysis[5] of gynecology textbooks published in the United States from 1943 to 1973. We were interested in textbooks because they provide the "official" gynecologic perspective of female sex role and sexuality and also because new practitioners, through reading these books, are trained to hold the same values and beliefs.

Our examination of twenty-seven textbooks revealed, with few exceptions, a persistent paternalistic and sometimes condescending attitude on the part of the doctor toward his female patient. Women were portrayed as most appropriately fitting into traditional sex roles: anatomically destined for motherhood, they were fulfilled as people only by reproducing, mothering, and attending to their husbands. Female sexuality was thus quantitatively and qualitatively misrepresented. There was also a tendency to regard the husband's role in marital and sexual matters as more important than the wife's. In short, gynecologists' values and beliefs, in the main, legitimated sex-role stereotypes.

For example, in the 1940s, when World War II gave women the opportunity to move into the labor force, one author, Willard Cooke, was moved to write "The very recent widening of the sphere of feminine activities, with the assumption of the male function of protection and maintenance, has led to a further weakening of the reproductive urge, resulting in the modern 'smart' type — sexless, frigid, self-sufficient."[6] Even in the 1970s gynecologists celebrated traditional women and castigated, in psychiatric terms, nontraditional women. One contended that "an emotionally healthy married woman will welcome pregnancy as a step toward maturity. The reasons for not wanting a child usually betray an underlying ambivalence toward the feminine role. They may be expressions of unconscious anxiety, conflict or inadequacy."[7] We consistently found gynecologists defining what the female role should be in terms of their own values and then labeling as emotionally unstable those women who sought fulfillment in other roles.

Biases were also evident in their discussions of female sexuality. In the 1940s, before the work of Kinsey and Masters and Johnson, women tended to be portrayed as relatively sexless and frigid. Female orgasms were believed to be less intense and pleasurable than the male variety. The true expression of sexualty for women was to be found in reproduction and motherhood. For example:

> The fundamental biologic factor in women is the reproductive urge of motherhood balanced by the fact that sexual pleasure is entirely secondary or even absent . . . One of the commonest problems presented for solution by the gynecologist is the vast and fundamental difference between the sexes in regard to sexual appetite. Women with their almost universal relative frigidity are apt to react to the marital relationship in one of three ways. (a) They submit philosophically to their husbands . . . (b) they submit rebelliously as a matter of duty . . . (c) they rebel completely and through refusal try to force the husband to adapt himself to their own scale of appetite.[8]

Male sexuality was perceived differently. Cooke states, "Biologically, for the preservation of the race, the male is created to fertilize as many females as possible and hence is given an infinite appetite and capacity for intercourse."[9] Here was the source of the chasm between the sexes: the male in a constant quest to impregnate as many females as possible, for the good of the race; the female, paradoxically, trying to avoid pregnancy in spite of her overpowering reproductive and maternal "instinct."

In the 1940s and 1950s most females were thought to be frigid, but rather than deal with the conditions that gave rise to the supposed situation, doctors directed treatment toward making the marital bed more comfortable for the male in order to preserve the marital relationship. From a 1952 text we learned:

> Unfortunate marital situations frequently arise because of the husband's resentment at the wife's sexual unrespon-

> siveness . . . It is good advice to recommend to the woman the advantage of innocent simulation of sex responsiveness, and as a matter of fact many women in their desire to please their husbands learned the advantage of such innocent deception.[10]

In the 1950s, with Alfred Kinsey's *Sexual Behavior in the Human Female,*[11] women did begin to receive some limited recognition as sexual beings. However, we found that when the researchers presented views of female sexuality radically different from that held by gynecologists, they were generally ignored. The reports were used selectively. Findings that reinforced old stereotypes were repeated, but the revolutionary findings significant for women received no notice. For example, one often finds in the textbooks that the male sets the sexual pace in marital coitus, but nowhere is it mentioned that women are multiorgasmic, a Kinsey finding, confirmed by William Masters and Virginia Johnson, that raises questions concerning the stronger male sex drive.

Though Kinsey is not usually credited with the discovery of women's capacity for multiple orgasm, he debunked the myth of the vaginal orgasm. He supplied anatomical evidence of the lack of surface nerve endings in the upper vagina and concluded that the vaginal orgasm was a "physical and physiological impossibility for nearly all females." Sensation, he averred, was primarily in the clitoris.

More recent works, such as Sherfey's *The Nature and Evolution of Female Sexuality,*[12] state that only the lower third of the vagina is sensitive, but that the thrusting action of the penis in intercourse activates clitoral nerve endings. "With maturation, the erotogenic zone of the lower third of the vagina does not supplant the clitoral zone; it must be assimilated with the entire clitoral-labial complex into a single functional structure."

This finding should have put an end to the Freudian dictum that the clitoral orgasm, induced by masturbation or manipulation, is an immature response, and the vaginal orgasm, achievable only through heterosexual intercourse, is the only mature sexual response for women. But in spite of Kinsey we frequently found textbooks from the fifties and sixties making definitive statements on female sexuality, such as:

> Investigators of sexual behavior distinguish between clitorial and vaginal orgasms, the first playing a dominant role in childhood sexuality and in masturbation and the latter in the normal mature and sexually active women . . . The limitation of sexual satisfaction to one part of the external genitalia is apparently due to habit and aversion to normal cohabitation.[13]

Another significant Kinsey finding had to do with the speed of sexual response in the female when the clitoris was manipulated. The average was found to be a few seconds under four minutes, with 45 percent of the sample achieving orgasm in under three minutes. Thus Kinsey concluded, "It is true that the average female responds more slowly than the average male in coitus but this seems to be due to the ineffectiveness of usual coital technique."

Our study did not find gynecologists suggesting coital technique be improved. Rather, we found statements such as:

> Some women are truly frigid . . . Psychic factors operate at the level of the cerebral cortex to inhibit the translation of sexual stimuli into pleasurable response. Unless there is a true aversion to sex the marital relations may proceed without disturbing either partner.[14]

In the early 1960s reports began to flow from the laboratories of Masters and Johnson.[15] These findings seem to have had more impact on the medical field than did Kinsey's, perhaps because Masters and Johnson's methods involved scientific observation under controlled laboratory conditions. Their findings reinforced Kinsey's by adding a physiological analysis of sexual response; for example, in the detailed description of the four phases of the response cycle. Though Masters and Johnson, like Kinsey, usually were not directly quoted in gynecology texts, there was some indirect influence. By 1967 most texts dropped the vaginal orgasm theory and began suggesting manipulation of the clitoris as part of foreplay.

The image of female sexuality had changed subtly in the texts. By the late 1960s women were no longer viewed as frigid but were allowed to enjoy sex in a self-limited and passive fashion. In 1967 Thomas Jeffcoate wrote, "An important feature of sex desire in the man is the urge to dominate the woman and subjugate her to his will; in the woman acquiescence to the masterful takes a high place."[16] The function of sex for women, however, was still perceived as being primarily for procreation: "During pregnancy the woman rarely has much sex desire because the fundamental object of coitus has been achieved and her mind is centered on the fetus in utero."[17] Even by 1970 we continued to find gynecologists identifying with the husband and the male role in marital and sexual matters. For example:

> The frequency of intercourse depends entirely upon the male sex drive . . . The bride should be advised to allow her husband's sex drive to set their pace and she should attempt to gear hers satisfactorily to his. If she finds after several months or years that this is not possible, she is advised to consult her physician as soon as she realizes there is a real problem. In assuming this role of follow the leader, however, she is cautioned not to make her sexual relations completely passive . . . She may be reminded that it is unsatisfactory to take a tone-deaf individual to a concert.[18]

Attitudes and beliefs like those revealed in this study are important because they serve as the background against which medical decisions are made. It is true that the attitudes of obstetrician-gynecologists who write textbooks cannot be applied to the whole profession, but the textbooks may be used as a source of authoritative information, especially when other forms of sex education are conspicuously missing in training.

Psychiatrist Harold Lief[19] of the Tulane University School of Medicine is noted for research that revealed the inadequacy of physicians in the treatment of sexual problems. For example, a

1959 study found that half of the medical students and a fifth of the faculty at five medical schools believed masturbation was a frequent cause of mental illness. Lief concluded:

> Few [physicians] know enough and fewer still have been adequately trained in the practical, clinical management of sexual problems. Worst of all, too many physicians still share with their patients the very misconceptions and misplaced inhibitions that give rise to sexual problems in the first place.[20]

In 1965, the AMA issued a mandate requiring medical schools to provide some type of "appropriate learning experience for physicians in the area of counseling related to sexual attitudes and behavior." The success of these programs is questionable. Pauline Bart[21] points out that the two departments most frequently responsible for sex education are, ironically, psychiatry and gynecology, the two disciplines that have been most criticized by feminists for their sexist ideologies and their sexist treatment of women patients.

The AMA edict on sexual education had not affected resident education at Elite or Mass. During my period of observation, neither institution offered instruction on female sexuality (though Elite planned to initiate a program the following year). Residents stated that the board qualifying examinations of the American College of Obstetricians and Gynecologists contained only a few superficial questions on sexuality, from which they inferred that the subject was not important. When asked where they acquired their knowledge of human sexuality, answers ranged from *Playboy* magazine to the army. Only a few had read even parts of Masters and Johnson.

In spite of this, the majority of residents believed sexual counseling was an important part of an obstetrician-gynecologist's work. A few residents indicated they would refer women with sexual problems elsewhere, but most expected to provide counseling personally, in spite of their acknowledged lack of information.

[Q. Do you feel adequate to give sexual counseling?]
No, I'm going to do it anyway and somehow I'm going to figure it out. Back in medical school we did have a brief, maybe two or three sessions . . . He [faculty member] was telling us how to give sexual counseling but that was only for a brief period and that's when I realized that was the only time that anybody ever talked to me about anything like that. Nobody ever talks about it here . . . I haven't really been trained in it. Hopefully somewhere I will get the training; I don't know where or how. (Interview, Elite.)

I think that half the problems you see in your office can be solved with sexual counseling.
[Q. Have you had any courses?]
No, but I will do some reading. (Interview, Mass.)

[Q. Do you think you will be able to give sexual counseling?]
Yes, I think so.
[Q. Where will your knowledge come from?]
Reading.
[Q. Have you read Masters and Johnson?]
No, but I saw them on TV. I don't agree with him 100 percent. You see a patient that has a sex problem, you have to make sure she doesn't have any disease first of all. The rest is 95 percent psychological problems, so you have to listen to them, let them talk and you can help. (Interview, Mass.)

Lack of sexual education in obstetrician-gynecologists may create other problems. A detailed 1969 study of sexual experience and anxiety among 397 male medical students[22] found that 42 percent felt less knowledgeable in sexual matters than other college graduates, and almost all, 91.5 percent, thought they were poorly prepared to counsel patients on sexual matters. In some cases their lack of specific information on human sexuality produced guilt and anxiety. For example, 10 percent of the medical students believed they masturbated excessively, evidently unaware that there is a normal wide range of masturbatory behavior among males. Of equal significance was the finding that even students who displayed strong feelings of personal sexual confidence and who had very active sexual lives experienced, like their less practiced and confident colleagues, a high level of sexual anxiety in their role as physician. Most important, the authors of the study concluded that sexual anxiety appreciably interferes with professional objectivity.

> More than a third of the students thought that ". . . the average student may be so uncomfortable while examining erotic areas that he may neglect to examine these organs . . ." and a sixth believed that staff doctors were susceptible to the same neglect. About three-fifths thought that ". . . the nervousness they experienced during their intimate contact with patients prevented them from being as effective as they might have been communicating with their patients . . ." and two-fifths were hampered in their thinking about differential diagnosis and management of their patients.[23]

These figures represent subjective responses, not actual behavior, leading the authors to suggest that objective interference may be even greater and that professional behavior is significantly affected by sexual anxiety.

Although the responses of professionally inexperienced medical students cannot be applied to relatively more experienced residents, it is nonetheless true that because obstetrician-gynecologists handle the erotically linked areas of the opposite sex, their work has the potential to be somewhat more anxiety-provoking than the work of other specialists. At the least, obstetrician-gynecologists are forced to confront these anxieties in a way other kinds of physicians may be able to avoid.

Information about sexual anxiety is difficult to elicit in face-to-face interviews. However, several residents volunteered information that closely paralleled the data on medical students. One departing resident, who planned to specialize in endocrinology and infertility, explained his embarrassment at discussing certain aspects of sexuality:

> [Q. Have you had any courses on sexuality?]
>
> No, any counseling I might provide would come from some kind of feelings that I have about it . . . On the other hand, I think many of us are hung up on sex and even though I would say that I am not, there probably are things that I would feel uncomfortable talking about. (Interview, Elite.)

A fourth-year resident made the following observation about the ritual connected with a pelvic exam and particularly about the physician's use of gloves:

> We have a nurse in the room, number one, you have a patient with her clothes on and a sheet, she doesn't have to be completely nude and you do a pelvic with gloves on. (Laugh.)
>
> [Q. I have seen many pelvics but I never considered the significance of the glove.]
>
> If you don't wear gloves, it is much more provocative.
>
> [Q. I always thought that was to prevent infection.]
>
> Infect, what you going to infect? The vagina is a dirty part of the body; what are you going to infect? (Interview, Elite.)

Another resident spoke of the way in which he was taught to control body language that might be interpreted as provocative:

> . . . We are taught that when we sit with a patient, we should never sit like this [he spread apart his legs]. It is too suggestive. We should sit with our feet together. (Interview, Mass.)

At Elite and Mass, although breast examinations were supposed to be part of all routine examinations, residents did them only sporadically; more often than not patients' breasts were not examined. In part, this can be explained by the clinic structure, which necessitates brief encounters with large numbers of women. Also, since residents cannot operate on disease found in the breast (it belongs to general surgery) as they can pathology located in the pelvis, they found it personally expedient to exclude this part of the examination. One resident, however, suggested the situation may, in part, be due to anxiety over examination of the breast:

> One thing I am going to mention because I think that it might be useful to you . . . the one exam that I do now with more facility and less consideration, one exam that comes close to having some social overtones that I have come of late to form my own defenses against is the breast exam.
>
> [Q. I have noticed most exams in the clinic don't include breast exams.]
>
> It's mostly expediency in the clinic, that's for sure. But there have been a number of times — like I say, I am just becoming a little more comfortable. For some reason in the past, I have attached much more sexual overtone to the breast exam than to doing a pelvic exam but recently it is better.
>
> [Q. Do you think that might be why it isn't done? The residents feel uncomfortable?]
>
> Part, I'm sure, is. That and, and I'll never know, but for expediency's sake in many cases, it is easy to overlook it, to ignore it. (Interview, Elite.)

During their training residents acquired the ability to objectify the erotically linked areas of the female body, in part by depersonalizing their interaction with the patient. Techniques such as the use of a drape during examination were (and are) used not just to protect the sensitivity of the woman but to protect the physician as well. Not only were personal feelings of sexual anxiety and embarrassment controlled, but clear boundaries between work and private life were maintained. Boundaries were important, because female patients not only "turned on" the residents but turned them off as well. As one resident stated, "A lot of those girls are pains in the neck and don't smell very good." (Interview, Elite.) Several residents who had pregnant wives explained that they did not want to be present for the deliveries because they wanted to avoid making an association between their wives and the women who were patients.

> My wife is three months' pregnant and she is going to see one of my colleagues in the clinic and he will deliver her and I don't want to be there except in the hospital. I trust the guy like I trust myself and that's it. I like to think my wife is a little different than my patients. (Interview, Mass.)

One resident explained the extent to which he maintains sexual boundaries:

> I think it is just completely impersonal, the vaginal exam. You know we do that every day; it's just like absolutely zero. You know you could be stark naked and I could do a pelvic on you and I wouldn't think anything of it. On the other hand, if you were out on the beach with a skimpy bathing suit on and I drove by, I would think, boy she is a pretty good-looking girl. You know, I think just being in the office, you just do it and that's it. There is no sexual connotation . . . I think most of it is very simple because most women aren't gorgeous, good-looking, and have terrific figures. A lot of them are fat, fifty, and disgusting. You know they are just fat and sexually you aren't attracted to them to begin with, much less when doing a pelvic exam on them.
>
> And even people that are average or good-looking . . . I would rather see somebody in clothes than naked on the table . . . the other thing is, you do it every day. It's not

> like you are in high school trying to get your first hand in a girl's bra. It's not something new; you do it fifty times a day. You know anything that you do fifty times a day isn't going to be a turn-on . . . Even if I have just done a total vulvectomy, with tubes out of everywhere, you know, it's just like boom, boom, you are out of there and into something else. (Interview, Mass.)

Depersonalization is an inevitable consequence of forcing attention away from the individual in medical interaction so that only the problem remains. Like other physicians, residents at Mass and Elite believed their interaction with patients had to be impersonal and objective, and socialization was incomplete until the resident was able to accomplish with ease the transition from person to problem.

> Well, I used to think that it [pelvic exam] was a problem when I was in college but it doesn't seem to be a problem anymore. I don't know why. To me it really doesn't seem sexual, although it is absolutely sexual; it doesn't seem that way. It doesn't seem threatening. It used to . . . In the same way listening to the chest doesn't seem like anything anymore. (Interview, Elite.)

Insofar as a physician's sexual education is related not only to the knowledge necessary for adequate patient counseling but to the reduction of his sexual anxiety and to ease in practitioner-client interaction, it would seem that some form of sexual education would be of basic importance for residents in obstetrics and gynecology, whose work is most intimately involved in sexual matters.

Learning Not to Care

One criticism of surgical training in general is that the caring aspect of healing is largely peripheral to the work for which a surgeon has been prepared. Since surgical residents see themselves as trainees in surgery and not in "bedside doctoring," they expect to learn the techniques of human relations after they enter private practice. As a result, a surgeon enters practice without caring skills.[24]

The same situation existed in the obstetrics-gynecology residency programs at Mass and Elite. The paradox, however, became very evident here because an obstetrician-gynecologist's work is different from that of a general surgeon. Unlike general surgeons, obstetrician-gynecologists have long-term relationships with patients who, for the most part, do not think of their physician as a surgeon but rather as someone who treats routine problems. Consequently, human relations skills are important and, especially in obstetrics, are an essential component of good patient care. Residents in both programs agreed about this.

> Well, I think part of prenatal care is giving a lot of support and judgment and so forth and to develop a nice relationship. That is what I think is really nice about ob-gyn, the fact that you are usually dealing with young people you can relate with — well, that you can talk with. And hopefully they will be able to talk to you and develop a nice, good, strong, personal relationship . . . You see, I think for me to continue to really like obstetrics and not to fall into the pattern of becoming disenchanted with obstetrics later in life, I think that the way I would have to practice is to get to know my patients really well. So that when I get up at 3:00 A.M. I'll say, "Gee, that's Mary Jane, she needs me there, and I really want to give my all." And if she has some kind of dysfunctional labor pattern, not be so quick to section her just because it is 3:00 A.M. and I don't want to stay up any longer. And that does happen. (Interview, Elite.)

> I suppose to be a physician, number one, you have to enjoy interpersonal relationships. You have to enjoy taking care of people, like people . . . you have to enjoy seeing people and taking care of people. You have to have

> a reasonable amount of patience to be an obstetrician. The obstetricians who constantly get into trouble are the ones who rush things. A very famous obstetrician once said that the obstetrician's single most important tool is a large cigar. You sit down and smoke it and let nature do her work. (Interview, Elite.)
>
> I think a good doctor is the one who cares about the people he is taking care of, who is willing to spend a lot of time — it has to do with interpersonal relations. (Interview, Elite.)

In spite of the belief that a personal relationship with a patient was a prerequisite for good obstetrical and gynecological care, attention to the human relations aspect of health care was not considered relevant in residency. This implies, first, that the poor are not entitled to considerate personal care and, second, that human relations skills can be quickly and easily acquired once the physician is in private practice and in competition for patients. It is also likely, however, that when training takes place in an atmosphere of uncaring, where patients are treated like objects to be exploited for their training value, the attitudes acquired become a permanent part of the physician's pattern of relating to people. Moreover, the training situation reinforces the cultural differences between physicians, who are predominantly white middle-class males, and patients, who are women, nonwhite, and poor. To understand fully how detrimental this situation is to the patient and the impact it makes on the developing physician's attitudes, it is necessary to understand the extent to which patients are used as teaching material within training hospitals.

Women as "Teaching Material"

Words are inadequate in describing what some people must endure to obtain health care. Readers who have anxiously waited with a sick child in the emergency room of a large public hospital, or who have spent hours in a clinic waiting room for two minutes with a resident who doesn't bother to use names or talk directly, already understand the feelings of degradation and alienation this type of health care produces.

Residents were always brief and impersonal. One typical routine gynecological examination at Elite began as the resident walked through the curtains saying, "Hello, dear." Sitting down as he read the chart, he asked the woman, "When was your last menstrual period? How many pregnancies have you had?" (Sometimes the patient would be asked to state her problem; other times it was just read off the chart.) Rising from the chair to insert the speculum so that he could get matter for a Pap smear and gonococcus culture, the resident ordered the woman to spread her legs and relax. A manual examination and a short explanation of the problem and treatment followed. The woman was asked if she had any questions and was told to dress and see the nurse while the resident wrote on the chart. Total time was about two minutes for an average patient with a minor problem. One resident told me, as he inserted the speculum, "I don't waste any time. I already have a diagnosis in mind. Patients get quick treatment." (Field Notes, Elite.)

Given the tone and pace of the clinic, many people would have difficulty asserting themselves sufficiently to ask a question. However, residents often interpreted patients' silence as an indication of hostility, stupidity, or ambivalence. Even if the patient was visibly upset, residents did not usually respond personally, as the following field notes indicate:

> The resident, two medical students, and I were in the examining room with a patient. This is her first pregnancy and it is very painful for her because she had polio as a child and is crippled. She appeared to be very upset, but no one tried to talk to her about it. At the end of the examination, the resident asked her if she had any questions and she said no but that she would like to talk to me. The others left the examining room and closed the

> curtain. I talked to her for about five minutes. She said that she is so afraid to have the baby that she wakes up at night crying. I tried to tell her what would happen in the delivery room and reassure her. I told her that she could have someone in the labor room with her. She said there was no one, absolutely no one, to be with her. (Field Notes, Elite.)

In cases such as this, a hospital social worker might be called on. In training hospitals, social workers counsel institutional patients on a wide variety of problems, from abortion to cancer. The result, however, is to lessen the opportunity for residents to learn such skills and develop a sense of responsibility and involvement with the patient.

The most striking example of our health care system was evident in the labor and delivery rooms at Elite. The contrast was heightened by the relatively small physical space in which two entirely different methods of childbirth existed side by side.

The private obstetrical patients of attending physicians were for the most part white, middle- or upper-middle-class, educated women who specifically sought Elite because the prevailing mode of delivery there was Lamaze childbirth. During my three months of observation in the labor and delivery rooms, at least 95 percent of private deliveries were of this type. Medical students were forbidden to touch private patients. Only residents were allowed to do the examinations necessary to determine labor progress. In short, private patients were afforded what the profession considered a deluxe obstetrical experience.

Institutional patients had a much different type of childbirth experience. During the period I observed, only one patient had a Lamaze delivery, and she was the wife of a student at the university associated with Elite. When I questioned residents about the obvious differences in delivery, they told me institutional patients couldn't afford Lamaze classes and that most of the women didn't have husbands to participate in the delivery process, anyway.

These rationalizations seemed to mask the real issue, which

was that if institutional patients were allowed to learn Lamaze techniques, the opportunity for residents to learn how to use forceps and other obstetrical techniques would be considerably reduced. Lamaze childbirth is supposed to be natural and is often accomplished without obstetrical intervention.

Besides determining the type of delivery, a patient's institutional status also affected her other experiences while in labor. The institutional patient was the woman on whom medical students and residents learned to judge dilation and effacement; sometimes a patient was subjected to three or four painful examinations at one time. Institutional patients were used as the material on which the students and residents learned the techniques for vaginal deliveries, forceps, episiotomies, and rotations.

Teaching hospitals, usually associated with medical schools, have always been organized primarily to train physicians. Since the health care system was never intended to provide the same services and care for the poor that is available to the middle class, teaching institutions are at liberty to structure services so that staff needs, rather than patient needs, are satisfied. Schedules and services at Elite and Mass were arranged to maximize the residents' opportunity to see pathology. The result for the patient was a lack of continuity in care. Residents might see a woman once or twice for prenatal care but would not be scheduled in the labor rooms during the period when she was to deliver. The most concerned and personal care developed on services where the resident had prolonged contact with the patient. At Elite this was most likely to occur in ward gynecology and at Mass in oncology. In both programs, the briefest encounters were in obstetrics. On the service where supportive, personal care was especially important, it was least likely to occur.

Residents were aware of the structural factors that limited their involvement with patients and often used them as an excuse for the type of care they delivered.

> It is difficult to arrange any residency program, I think, into one where you can handle patients effectively, with

economy of time and space, and have someone conduct almost a private practice; it's just not possible. Besides that, a residency program has to provide its residents with a cross-section of pathology and techniques and so on. It's just not that easy to accomplish.

[Q. Do you think this residency allows you to develop a good relationship with your patients?]

No, not at all, absolutely zero . . . When you first start residency, you have a limited amount of time, you are pushed and you learn, and you really become involved in your own training. Some people don't do this but I think the majority of people do. And also when you are in a big teaching hospital, you can't develop the personal relationship with patients. When I was chief of ob, which was in my third year, I had patients on the floor that I was following for long periods of time for various problems they had before they delivered, and I got to develop a real nice relationship with them over this period of time. So when it came time for them to deliver, I really felt I had to be there and had to be part of it. I was completely devoted to giving them the best possible care.

One of the big problems here is that there is no continuity in patient-doctor care. A patient may see me one week and I may not see her again for another five weeks, or I may have seen her on her first visit and not see her again until thirty-six weeks later or I may never see her again. I have no idea if my prenatal management was the correct thing. If she comes in and delivers a good baby, you get no feedback. You get feedback only if things go badly, if somebody screws up along the way. Same thing in the labor rooms; 95 percent of the time you are delivering someone that you have had no involvement with in their prenatal care. You don't know them, they are just a name, a body, they are delivering . . . There is no involvement with the patient and that's bad because I think later on that is a very important part of your practice. (Interview, Elite.)

In addition to the structural problems of institutional health care, the personal goals of many of the residents further reduced personal care. Residents believed their function in training was to acquire technical skill and judgment. The treatment patients received reflected this priority. The point is best illustrated by comparing the work performed by residents with that done by nurse-midwives.

At Mass, nurse-midwives (nurses with additional clinical training in ob-gyn) trained midwifery students and worked in the prenatal clinic, family planning clinic, and on the labor row, where they performed "normal deliveries." On their first visit to the prenatal clinic, patients were sorted into normal and high-risk categories. "Normals" were randomly assigned to nurse-midwives (who handled fewer cases than residents) or to residents. After her first visit with a nurse-midwife, the woman was asked if she wanted to continue her prenatal care with a nurse-midwife or if she preferred to see a doctor. According to clinic personnel and my own observations, the usual response was to request the continued services of a nurse-midwife. From this point on, the woman belonged to the midwifery service. When she came to the labor row, the woman was attended to and delivered by the nurse-midwife on duty.

Nurse-midwives were so obviously different in the way in which they treated and related to women that even residents noticed and commented on it:

> Well, one thing about the midwives is, I think that when a patient comes into the hospital, they like to have someone with them all the time, like that is one of the complaints we get on the labor row. A woman might be making progress and you understand that she is making progress, but she is just lying there having pains and is very apprehensive about it. But when a midwife follows the patient, she is there all the time, she holds her hand, she explains, she talks, and I think this is one of the main areas where medicine really falls short, the handholding. On the labor row I don't think that you can.

> [Q. Sometimes it is very busy, but sometimes it isn't?]
> Well, sometimes it isn't, but you have to be in the habit of handholding, it has to be part of your habit. (Interview, Mass.)

> The midwives spend a lot more time with patients . . . Residents say they don't have time but sometimes we have only two patients and more time, but we definitely don't spend as much time with the patients as the midwives do. The midwives look for a lot more things and they are a lot more precise about each thing than the residents are. The problem with that is they keep bringing things up that may be a problem but five times out of six it isn't a problem so they are just looking too hard for things to go wrong . . . They are very slow, they are very careful, they don't want to miss anything, and if the smallest thing is askew, they want to do something now. Sometimes they pick something up, true, but most of the time it's something that you really don't have to worry about. (Interview, Mass.)

A common argument against nurse-midwives' participation in childbirth has been that they are not able to recognize pathology, so they jeopardize good obstetrical care. However, research has indicated the opposite. In one controlled study, it was found that nurse-midwives were able to recognize deviations from normal in the obstetrical patient, would ask for medical consultation promptly, and could render safe, effective service themselves to about one third of a high-risk obstetrics population.[25]

In part, the difference between the way in which nurse-midwives and residents performed their work can be explained by the way each group defined its participation in childbirth and its function within the context of institutional health care. Midwives have traditionally defined their role in childbirth as assisting women in the natural process of giving birth. Modern nurse-midwives also provide well care and treat the routine conditions associated with the female reproductive function. Obstetrical residents, on the other hand, see themselves as physicians-in-training and institutional patients as the material on which technical skills can be practiced and judgment sharpened. Too, physicians view childbirth as a medical problem rather than a natural process. One attending physician at Mass, for example, was fond of telling residents that as long as there was a pregnant woman between the sheets there was a problem on the ward.

Because of their basically different orientations and roles in childbirth, nurse-midwives and residents emphasized different skills. In addition to the technical aspects of the usual vaginal deliveries, which both residents and midwives learned, residents were taught surgical-intervention procedures such as use of forceps and the cesarean section. Nurse-midwives, on the other hand, were taught to care for their clients, and human relations skills were stressed. An important part of the nurse-midwives' work involved sitting with their patients throughout the entire labor process, talking, explaining and giving support, teaching controlled breathing, and applying gentle abdominal massage. Midwifery instructors believed that women would experience fewer complications and have healthier babies if they were supported and comforted during labor. They often complained about medical students who, because they were not taught the caring aspect of childbirth, expected to be allowed to deliver the nurse-midwife's patients but refused to sit with them while they were in labor.

Residents argued that because they were responsible for all the complications on the labor row, they were too busy to give individual attention. But even when they had only a single patient in labor, they spent no additional time with her. As the resident quoted before observed, "You have to be in the habit of handholding" in order to give that kind of care.

Residents and midwifery instructors had the same function on the labor row. Both were engaged in teaching students the technical aspects of routine deliveries, and neither had long-term relationships with the women they delivered. As with residents, the nurse-midwife on the labor row might not be the same person the woman had seen for most of her prenatal care. In spite of these similarities, residents and nurse-midwives interacted quite differently with women during delivery, as the following field notes indicate.

> One of the primary differences between a delivery conducted by a nurse-midwife and a resident's delivery appears to be in the interaction between the medical personnel and the woman delivering. The conversation in a resident's delivery is between himself and whoever is assisting him. Some of this can be explained as necessary teaching. However, in this delivery the nurse-midwife is also teaching, yet both instructor and student find time to talk to the woman. Unlike the resident, in the case of the nurse-midwife there is constant communication between the two, which begins when the nurse-midwife performs the first step in a delivery: inserting two fingers into the vagina to feel the position of the baby. The nurse-midwife tells the woman what she is going to do and from that point on she explains every step in the process.
>
> In a few cases the resident may also explain the first step to the woman, but after that will say nothing to her until the baby is born, when he may tell her what sex it is. Therefore, in a resident's delivery the woman is out of touch with what is happening in her body, it is mystifying for her. Not only does the nurse-midwife explain what she is doing, but she gives her support, tells her that she is doing well, that she is a good patient, and when possible continues the gentle stroking begun during the labor process. At the moment of birth, the woman's head is held up so that she can see what is occurring. Residents never do this. The nurse-midwife immediately places the baby on the mother's stomach while cutting the cord. Residents hold the baby, cut the cord, and place him or her on a steel table for examination and eye drops. The nurse-midwife gives the newborn to the mother to hold, tells her

> what a beautiful baby she has and that she did very well. Residents never allow the woman to hold the baby and never comment on it except to say that it has the requisite number of fingers and toes.
>
> The nurse-midwife also tells the mother the infant's Apgar score. Residents never give women this information and indeed their patients wouldn't know what Apgar was. The nurse-midwife continues to chat with the woman while waiting for the placenta to separate. She then carefully checks the placenta, including the cord. Residents give the placenta a very cursory examination. During the delivery, the nurse-midwife calls the woman by her name. Residents use "dear," which is easier than learning a name. (Field Notes, Mass.)

In contrast to residents, nurse-midwives also performed their clinic work in a more personal manner. Nurse-midwives gave more thorough examinations. For example, they always included a breast examination as well as instruction, with the use of a rubber model, on self-examination. Nurse-midwives, unlike residents, always explained what they were doing and why, as well as teaching their patients about their bodies. Because the interaction was relaxed and friendly, as opposed to hurried and impersonal, the nurse-midwives' patients usually felt free to ask questions. In contrast, clinic nurses told me that the residents' patients often complained because they were told to "get dressed" before they could ask a question. In short, nurse-midwives informed and residents confused their patients.

Not only did nurse-midwives and residents differ in their orientation toward women's health care, resulting in an emphasis on different skills, but within the context of a training hospital the two groups had different goals. The first priority of nurse-midwives was to provide good care for women. The residents' top priority was to acquire training; obstetrics patients were simply means to this end. Patient treatment, in this case, was considerably affected by the perspectives and goals of those delivering the care.

In addition to the limitations imposed on personalized care by structural factors and training goals, there was an additional factor that influenced the manner in which residents related to their patients. Over and over, residents, especially at Elite, told me they disliked institutional patients. Especially in obstetrics, the young, unmarried black women and women who lost control during delivery were a source of scorn.

> I think it is very difficult to deal with the institutional patients that we are dealing with. I don't plan to have them in private practice. I don't plan to have a lot of fourteen- and fifteen-year-old girls that are pregnant in my office. (Interview, Elite.)

> I'm sure you have seen what we have here. We have a lot of young girls having their first baby, some fourteen, even twelve; they are scared to death. They scream and shout, they won't lie in bed, they pull out their IVs, they won't let you examine them, that kind of business. (Interview, Elite.)

> It's much nicer to have a nice gravida two or three that can verbalize all her problems to you rather than a gravida fourteen who can't even remember all their names let alone how much she weighed or where they were born. But that is my own upbringing. (Interview, Mass.)

> It's a lot easier to take care of somebody that you can relate to — uh — I suppose that living a relatively sheltered existence, at least in terms of the people that I came into contact with, I really didn't have any close contact with the kind of people that come to Elite clinic until I got here . . . There is no kick in delivering a thirteen-year-old-unmarried child of a third illegitimate child of her third illegitimate child. And there is no kick in seeing a lady who, you know, decided to say that her boyfriend raped her because she had a fight with him in a bar that night,

> and there is no kick in seeing a girl who comes in every week with PID. (Interview, Elite.)

> I think basically I don't like to deal with uneducated people. They are people that know it is going to hurt and just start yelling from the beginning. (Interview, Elite.)

> It will be a much closer relationship [with private patients] because most of the institutional patients, at least I'm not that overly concerned about them. If someone comes to the clinic, I'm not going to say "You are the one girl that I want to deliver and follow all through the pregnancy. When you go into labor, call me at the house and I'll be right over." (Interview, Elite.)

Residents admitted that women whom they disliked were not given the same care as those they favored.

> You know there are some people that you like and some people you can't stand. There is nothing wrong with that; everyone has it. If I like a patient, I will just automatically spend more time if I am busy or not busy. If somebody is over there screaming and raising hell, somebody that I don't like, they are just going to lay there. If something is wrong, fine, I will go see them, deliver them, make sure everything is all right. But I won't give that extra input that I would with somebody I got along with. (Interview, Mass.)

> It's a personality thing, and with the institutional patients, you don't have anything to say about it, you have to take care of them. If you don't like the patient and they don't like you, they don't get taken care of properly. (Interview, Elite.)

Sociologist Nancy Stoller Shaw[26] describes the dehumanization of maternity patients in her study of pregnancy and childbirth. She argues that two groups of factors affect the treatment patients receive: background (including ethnic heritage, marital status, education, income, age, number of children, and religion) and attitude (including plans for the child, weight control, and response to the staff). The closer the patient was to the staff in these matters, the better the treatment she received. The ideal patient from the staff's point of view was a white, married student in her early twenties having her first child, college educated, Protestant, with a temporarily low income but anticipated upper-middle-class status. She gained little weight, planned to keep her baby, and was classified as "pleasant." The patient who was liked least was black, separated, over thirty, with a large family supported by welfare. She gained weight, planned to give away her baby, and was classified as "dumb" or "hostile." Shaw states that patients who resembled the latter type were treated like animals, not persons. Residents, moreover, believed these patients got what they deserved.

Large class and sex differences, like those between white, upper-middle-class, male residents and poor or working-class, minority women, can be expected to produce difficulty in communication. They should not, however, be allowed to result in the dehumanized treatment that institutional patients sometimes received.

> Dr. P., the attending in the clinic today, and I discovered that we had been at the university at the same time and this opened up the conversation. He asked me if he could be perfectly candid. Up to this point I have been observing in the clinics. He told me to wait until I got to labor and delivery — that was where I would really see a lot. He said that I should especially watch the difference between the delivery of private and institutional patients. He said that I should also watch the difference between first-, second-, third-, and fourth-year residents and how they develop "finesse." Then he added that some never learn it. He said that I would be shocked at some of what I would see and that some residents were just cruel and cause all kinds of unnecessary pain and suffering, and he

> shivered. I asked what they did in a case like that and he said that they talk to them but that doesn't mean that they will change. (Field Notes, Elite.)
>
> In the labor lounge, I spent some time talking to a couple of nurses. One said that I would probably be interested in the way residents treated institutional patients. She said that though she felt she shouldn't say it, she believed the residents were mean to institutional patients. (Field Notes, Elite.)
>
> I talked for a while to the ward clerk* who is black. She works on the floor where all the obstetrical patients are housed before and after delivery. She wanted to know what I was doing and I told her. She said that perhaps I could answer a question for her. She wanted to know why the residents are the way they are. She said they treat the institutional patients as if they were "less than human." She repeated several times that she just couldn't understand why they treat the institutional patients as if they were less than human. (Field Notes, Elite.)
>
> I talked to a young woman who was having her second baby at Elite. She said that she wished it was over because "they let you suffer down there and the doctors are mean." I asked her what she meant and she said she knows that the patients who pay get treated better than the ones who are on aid. I asked her how she knew and she said that one of her friends had a baby as a paying customer and that she was treated much differently. (Field Notes, Elite.)

At the beginning of my observation period at Elite, residents made an effort to conceal from me the way some patients were treated. However, as the field work progressed and my presence became familiar on the wards, some of the residents began to talk to me about their own behavior. A first-year resident said:

* Employee on each hospital unit who performs clerical duties and often acts as receptionist.

> I think that they [institutional patients] are not treated very well at all. I think residents make very little effort to relate to these patients, even myself. I don't, even though I am conscious of the error . . . The institutional patients can either be very demanding or they can be extremely passive. I'm not sure why they should be either one way or the other. Some of these patients really bother me. I mean why are they so passive; either they have very little motivation in terms of themselves, or they don't seem to care very much about anything, whether they have the baby or don't have the baby . . . Some of the institutional patients are hostile. They probably have a right to be because of the way they are being treated. I don't know, I have thought about it; it's a difficult problem. I've read about it; it's a sickness throughout the United States. I don't know what to do about it, I really don't. (Interview, Elite.)

At the end of another interview, after the tape recorder was turned off, a resident told me the following:

> We started talking about the way he had answered some of the questions and he told me that since he knew there was a tape recorder going, he wasn't going to put his foot in his mouth. He said that he hadn't answered some of the questions honestly. The reason for this, he said, was that he was ashamed of the way he really felt because he wasn't giving good health care. He said that when he gets a screaming, hysterical fourteen-year-old in labor he is as likely to walk out and let her suffer as he is to do anything about it. He said that he knows that it is wrong and he is ashamed of it and embarrassed and he doesn't think it is proper patient care.
>
> However, he said that he cannot relate to institutional patients and that he has trouble feeling any kind of sympathy for them. He feels very strongly that personal care and a good relationship are very important for a private

> physician and he will work to achieve them. But as far as the institutional population goes, that is not a consideration. (Paraphrased from an untaped portion of Interview, Elite.)*

In the labor and delivery rooms at Elite, the teen-agers were the most vulnerable patients. Numerous painful pelvic examinations were done on institutional patients, sometimes four or five at a time to provide training for medical students, who were, by rule, not allowed to touch private patients. These examinations were sometimes done while the woman was having a contraction, thus increasing her pain, or after the membranes had ruptured, thus increasing the danger of infection. During these examinations, if the woman squirmed or yelled, she was told in an angry, authoritarian voice to behave or she would not be helped. Frightened teen-agers often would reach out to touch a hand, but if the hand belonged to a resident it was usually jerked away abruptly, with an accompanying admonition to behave. Another form of punishment was the withholding of pain medication; when patients complained of being in pain, they were told they were not in pain. The processes occurring in their bodies were never explained to them, nor were patients addressed except to receive orders. Patients' progress and problems were discussed among staff as if the patients were not present.

The behavior established in the labor room was carried over to the delivery room. The normal oral banter between patients and staff that took place in private deliveries was not extended to institutional patients, with whom conversation was limited to commands. When private patients, overcome with pain, lost control, they were reassured by the staff and told that they had a right to scream. When the delivery was over, they were always

* In the days following this interview, the resident hinted several times that he had said too much. Once when I was going with him to watch him do workups, he told me that he would rather that I didn't watch because he was ashamed of the sloppy job he does.

told they had done a good job. When institutional patients screamed, they were orally assaulted and strapped down.

Private patients were allowed to have their husbands in the delivery room to comfort and support them and to ensure courteous treatment by the staff, but institutional patients were not permitted the same right. Unlike a private patient, an institutional patient was never given her newborn to hold after delivery. Instead, the infant was placed in a warming chamber across the room and out of the mother's view. The infant of a private patient, after being held, was placed in a warming chamber and rolled to the mother's side.

At Mass, though patient care was hurried, impersonal, and sometimes inept, I did not observe residents engage in cruel behavior, though I was told stories about past occurrences. Because Mass was a public institution and could turn no one away, it was known as the city "dumping ground" and tended to get more patients with "undesirable" characteristics. Thus, I had expected to find the treatment of patients even worse than at Elite. This was not the case for several reasons.

At Mass, there was less class difference between residents and patients than at Elite, and a larger number of Mass residents were black, Spanish-speaking, or female. These factors do not always result in a "consciousness of kind," but they do facilitate, to some degree, understanding and communication.

There was also a substantial difference in the supporting personnel in the two institutions. At Mass, the presence of nurse-midwives on the labor row appeared to have a positive effect on patient care. Not only did nurse-midwives present an example to other staff of how women in childbirth should be treated; they attended to many of the women personally. At Elite the discriminatory treatment of institutional patients was heightened by the ever-present contrast with the way in which private patients were treated. An observer was constantly confronted with visible proof of the inequality in our health care system.

There were other differences in hospital personnel. At Elite, black workers were engaged mostly in nonskilled, low-level positions, and the individuals in professional and supervisory positions were, for the most part, white. At Mass, the majority of nonphysician staff, including professional and supervisory, were black and in many cases came from the same backgrounds and even the same neighborhoods as their patients. In contrast to Elite, the nursing staff at Mass appeared to identify more closely with patients than with physicians. Mass residents, in fact, spoke about the "lack of respect" they received from the staff. The staff were also able to exert some control because Mass was chronically understaffed, so if nurses chose not to cooperate with a particular resident, his job became considerably more difficult. This suggests that the staff at Mass, in contrast to Elite, provided a check, or at least a buffer, against inappropriate behavior on the part of residents.

Finally, the two institutions were different. Mass was an institution constantly caught in the crossfire of city politics, with various interest and advocate groups serving a "watchdog function." Because of the political pressure on the institution, policies that attempted to protect patient rights had to be initiated. I was impressed, for example, to find signs in examining rooms on the Mass gynecology wards warning staff that no patient was to undergo more than three pelvic examinations.* A copy of "The Patient's Bill of Rights" was posted on all the wards, and there were official means for patients to make known their grievances. The most frequently used were the social workers, who spent a great deal of time on the wards. Several times during my observations, residents were admonished for speaking incorrectly to patients. Further, the large open wards and labor rooms at Mass provided visibility, so actions were easily monitored. Though Mass had other problems, an attempt was made to protect patients against some of the abuses of the poor in institutionalized medicine. At Elite, these issues were largely ignored. The contrast between Elite and Mass points to the insufficiency of a system in which the only control on physi-

* Since pelvic exams were done for teaching purposes, a woman could be subjected to any number, depending on how many medical students, interns, and residents were present and the amount of interest her problem aroused.

cians' behavior is professional self-regulation. This issue is discussed at length in Chapter VII.

Many factors in residency combined to retard the development of caring. Residents were not encouraged to treat women in a positive or supportive way. No attempt was made to understand the problems and stresses of concern to women in general or to patients in particular. Residents may have believed that private patients were entitled to different treatment, but it is difficult to alter attitudes and behavior patterns acquired through years of training. Even if they did change, the poor would not be compensated.

Residents often said that "the telephone book is full of doctors." Obstetrician-gynecologists depend on word-of-mouth referrals from patients, and residents were aware that paying customers would not return to or recommend an obstetrician who treated them the way poor women were treated. In this respect, it is interesting to note how intricately the profit motive is linked to patient care. Socialized medicine, I was often warned, would result in treatment for everyone similar to what is currently reserved for the poor. It is not suggested that all obstetrician-gynecologists are motivated by profit, but profit is a major consideration for many.

> You serve a different purpose in private practice. You are a father image or a psychiatrist or a friend, or something like that. Here we don't give that kind of service to the patients; they don't expect it. A lot of what you do in private practice is that, plus figure out what you are going to do with your money, trying to make money. You are involved in different goals. (Interview, Elite.)

Many physicians are unable to effect more than a superficial change once out of training.

> Well, some people do it overnight. It's something that some people think is expected of them, and it can be a very phony, insincere thing. You know it's part of the

> image you might have to project . . . People anticipate it and expect it. So you smile and you call them dolly, sweety, pumpkin, things like that, and you pat them on the behind and you sort of talk down to them and everything and — uh — it's all very superficial. (Interview, Elite.)

Physicians argue that they must maintain an emotionally neutral position if they are to dispense medical care properly. We have seen that physicians are not neutral and that value judgments that affect treatment are made. Sociologist Julius Roth[27] questions whether emotional neutrality is even a characteristic worth striving for in health care. He argues that the best care is given by those for whom the patient is a special case and suggests that, since it hasn't been possible to train physicians to care, loved ones should be trained to perform routine medical and hospital duties. It is certainly possible to involve loved ones to a greater degree as caretakers and as advocates for the sick. But this is not enough. Health care needs to be transformed into a system that gives the highest priority to patient needs.

Although training in obstetrics and gynecology focuses on surgery and other forms of treatment for acute and pathological conditions, the majority of problems that women bring to their physicians do not require these treatments. Still, residents were mainly interested in learning and doing surgery and had professional identities closely linked to the surgeon's role. A career oriented toward preventive care and well care was viewed as having less potential for advancement, profit, and satisfaction than a surgical or superspecialty career. Some of the skills expected in a woman's generalist, therefore, were de-emphasized or even ignored in training. This suggests that in obstetrics and gynecology the amount of surgery performed is due to more than an oversupply of surgeons. The interests of the profession conflict with the real health care needs of women. Surgeons, not generalists, are being trained to service a population with mostly everyday medical, nonsurgical, nonsuperspecialty problems. This situation is ripe for the proliferation of unnecessary operations. All of this needless interference with women's bodies is increasing the hazards of iatrogenesis, a term coined to refer to the damage caused by the medical care system, including such things as infections, overmedication, and the removal of healthy organs. Thus, women not only suffer from diseases and malfunctions of their reproductive organs but also from damages inflicted on them by physicians and the health care system.

Hysterectomy — A Case in Point

Several studies have shown a relationship between the number of surgeons in practice and the amount of surgery performed. In the United States, where there are twice as many surgeons in proportion to the population as in England and Wales, there is also twice as much surgery.[28] One study found that the rate of surgery in Kansas was dependent on the supply of surgeons and facilities in a region rather than on the incidence of disease.[29] Other research has shown that so many physicians are performing surgery that the work loads of specialists are modest, thus making it difficult for them to maintain their surgical skills.[30]

Surgery of all types is increasing in the United States. The annual rate of operations in 1973 was 89.5 per 1000 population; in 1974, the rate was 92.9 per 1000 population; and in 1975, the rate was an estimated 95.8 per 1000 population. Overall, the rate of surgery is growing four times faster than the population.[31]

Hysterectomies in particular head the list of operations that have increased over the past ten years. Evidence suggests the increase is traceable to attitudes and practices within obstetrics and gynecology — reflected in resident training — rather than to an increase in disease among women.

In the ten year period between 1960 and 1970, the birth rate declined from 118.0 to 66.7 per 1000 women aged 15 to 44. The average number of children born to a family dropped to 1.8 in 1975, compared to 3.7 in 1957. At the same time the birth rate was dropping, hysterectomies were increasing. Between 1970 and 1975 hysterectomies increased 24 percent. According to government statistics, in 1975, 725,000 hysterectomies were performed, compared to 685,000 tonsillectomies and 319,000 appendectomies.[32] Thus, the hysterectomy now surpasses the former top-ranking operations and is the most commonly performed major surgery for women. It is estimated that if the present rates continue, 50 percent of all women in the United States will have a hysterectomy by the age of 65.[33] Among all types of surgery, the hysterectomy was outnumbered only by 1.7 million dilation and curettages (D & Cs), also a gynecological procedure and one commonly used in abortion.

There is ample reason to believe many of these hysterectomies were unnecessary. A recent study of a second-surgical-opinion program in New York found that 43 percent of 384 recommended elective hysterectomies and 36 percent of 115 recommended elective dilation and curettages were not confirmed in a second opinion. Among recommended mandatory procedures, 21 percent of 94 hysterectomies and 20 percent of 136 dilation and curettages were not confirmed.[34] In another study, a group of researchers in Saskatchewan, Canada, observing that hysterectomies had increased 72.1 percent between 1964 and 1971 while the number of women over 15 had increased only 7.6 percent, analyzed the hysterectomies performed in several hospitals during 1970, 1973, and 1974. The rate of unjustified hysterectomies varied by hospital, but in one it was as high as 59 percent. Moreover, though the average rate of unjustified hysterectomies for all hospitals studied was 23.7 percent in 1970, the average rate in these hospitals dropped to 7.8 percent in 1974, when surgeons were aware that their work was being monitored.[35]

Interestingly, the increase in hysterectomies has not been uniformly distributed over the female population. The number of hysterectomies performed for insured women is double that for uninsured. In prepaid health plans, where unnecessary surgery is not profitable, the rates are as much as a fourth lower than in fee-for-service plans. Hysterectomies are performed two and a half times as often in the United States as in England,[36] where medicine is socialized. Some increase in the rate of hysterectomies performed may be attributed to improved cancer detection measures, but the variation in these rates and the rate of unconfirmed procedures indicate that other factors are responsible for the observed increase.

Contrary to belief, relatively few of the hysterectomies are performed to treat cancer. In 1975, the executive director of the American College of Obstetricians and Gynecologists estimated that 15 percent of hysterectomies were done for cancer, 30 percent for noncancerous fibroids, 35 percent for pelvic relaxation or prolapse, and 20 percent for sterilization.[37] Ignoring sterilizations for the moment, it should be noted that surgical indications for benign disease such as fibroids and pelvic relaxation are a matter of clinical judgment. For example, fibroids (referred to by residents as the Cadillac of gynecology) are benign tumors frequently found in the female uterus. They are often small and asymptomatic and, left alone, can disappear without surgical intervention. Whether the uterus should be removed in such cases is a matter of judgment, and a physician's judgment can be influenced by bias.

Age is one factor in such bias. A study published in the *American Journal of Obstetrics and Gynecology*[38] noted that the average age of women having abdominal hysterectomies was 43.2 years, and 49.9 years for vaginal hysterectomy. My own observations indicate that young or reproductive women were less likely to be told they needed a hysterectomy for benign disease than were older women, past childbearing years, or women with either completed families or large families. This is linked to the fact that many obstetrician-gynecologists see no purpose in the woman's keeping her uterus after childbearing is completed.

The degree of surgical intervention can also be influenced by the suspected extent of the woman's sexual activity. An extreme is the practice of sewing the vagina closed (the LeFort operation) for a slipped or prolapsed uterus. As one textbook put it, this would be done "only in the elderly spinster or widow."[39]

In the late sixties, as birth rates began to decline, a new trend appeared in the profession. Obstetrician-gynecologists started substituting as a method of sterilization the hysterectomy, which is major surgery, for the tubal ligation, which is minor surgery. At the Los Angeles County University of Southern California Medical Center, during the period 1968 to 1970, the number of elective hysterectomies for a stated primary purpose of sterilization increased 742 percent, and the total number of all types of sterilization procedures increased 282 percent.[40]

Indicative of this trend, the 1970 edition of the popular *Novak's Textbook of Gynecology* cautiously stated that, though the authors were not making a case for "prophylactic hysterectomy [removal of a nondiseased uterus for the purpose of preventing conception], it should not be construed as callous if many gynecologists feel that, in the woman who has completed her family, the uterus is a rather worthless organ."[41] But by the time the 1975 edition of the textbook was published, the authors' position on prophylactic hysterectomy had changed to approval: "Within the last five years there has been increasing enthusiasm among many gynecologists for hysterectomy, especially vaginal, as an elective method of sterilization."[42] The authors note that there is greater morbidity and mortality and longer and more expensive hospitalization with a hysterectomy than with a tubal ligation, but they write, "Many gynecologists feel very strongly that vaginal hysterectomy is much preferred over tubal ligation, and can advance the following rather convincing arguments."[43] These include an approximate 2 percent pregnancy rate following tubal ligation and the observation that some women who have tubal ligations subsequently have other types of pelvic surgery. The authors note, furthermore, that "menstruation is a nuisance to most women, and if this can be abolished without impairing ovarian function, it would probably be a blessing to not only the women but to their husbands."[44] Thus they conclude, ". . . There seems definitely a trend in this community, as well as the country as a whole, for this to be the procedure of choice. Obviously this should be qualified by the fact that the surgery be done by a competent, well-trained gynecologist."[45]

Some obstetrician-gynecologists recommend not only prophylactic hysterectomy but removal of the total reproductive tract, including Fallopian tubes and ovaries, thereby reducing estrogen production and causing menopause. J. B. Skelton asserted to a gathering of the American College of Obstetricians and Gynecologists that:

> the time has come for us as members of this College to recognize and recommend prophylactic elective total hysterectomy and bilateral salpingo-oophorectomy [removal of Fallopian tubes and ovaries] after completion of childbearing as proper preventive medicine in obstetrics and gynecology . . . What benefits are derived from this operation? (1) It almost completely eliminates the occurrence of that feared killer of women, cancer of the uterus and ovaries. (2) It assures women of absolute voluntary sterilization. (3) It reduces the performance of multiple gynecologic operations each carrying some risk. (4) It relieves women of unpleasant and uncomfortable monthly bleeding. (5) It allows smooth maintenance therapy with feminizing hormones, eliminating bothersome cyclic variations, tensions, and emotionally altered states which affect the woman's world. (6) It decreases the frequency of unpleasant, humiliating pelvic exams and tests and allows better utilization of available health personnel, facilities, and time. And all of this can be achieved with one single operation. *Seldom in life do we risk so little to gain so much.*[46] (Emphasis mine.)

Do women really risk so little? A 1975 study by Cornell University Medical College indicated that 787,000 hysterectomies were performed in 1975, resulting in 1700 deaths. Surgery was unnecessary in an estimated 22 percent of the cases, resulting in 374 avoidable deaths.[47] In addition, a number of studies have shown that morbidity is much greater with a hysterectomy than it is with a tubal ligation.[48] For example, one study found operative complications in 51 percent of cesarean section hysterectomies and 22 percent of elective vaginal hysterectomies, but in only 1 percent of postpartum tubal ligations and 2 percent of elective abdominal tubal ligations.[49] The expense of a hysterectomy is four to five times greater than that of a tubal ligation, and recovery, only a few days for the latter procedure, is six weeks for a hysterectomy. Another study found that 42.7 percent of women undergoing vaginal hysterectomy experienced postoperative morbidity; the figure was only 1.5 percent for laparoscopic tubal ligation and 20.7 percent for abdominal tubal ligation.[50] (A laparoscope is an instrument similar in design to a periscope on a submarine. When it is inserted into the abdomen, the surgeon is able to view the female organs. By inserting another instrument, he is able to cauterize the tubes.) Observing that women are seldom advised of the relative dangers or complications of the two procedures, the Washington, D.C., Health Research Group states, "What is clear is that in many instances there is little evidence of informed consent by the patient and that these operations have been 'sold' to the public by surgeons in a manner not unlike many other deceptive marketing practices."[51]

These abuses are not confined to middle-class women. The rate of unneeded surgery on Medicare recipients has become so "intolerably high" that in November 1977, the Department of Health, Education, and Welfare announced it would begin to pay for second surgical opinions.[52] In fact, the thinking that condones unnecessary surgery is established in training, where residents learn that it is permissible to perform unnecessary surgery on the poor in order to get experience. The Health Research Group concluded:

> Surgical teaching programs are having increasing difficulty finding subjects to learn on because they greatly depend on the availability of ward or indigent patients and with increased third-party payments, the number of such patients is shrinking. As a consequence, residents in many city hospitals have done more "selling."[53]

There are other dangers connected with the hysterectomy. Surgeons often remove healthy ovaries as well as the uterus, arguing that it is a precaution against ovarian cancer, which is difficult to detect — but also rare. When the ovaries are removed, estrogen production is diminished, and as a result some women experience such menopausal symptoms as hot flashes. To prevent these symptoms from occurring, whether through natural or surgically induced menopause, physicians have prescribed estrogen replacement therapy (ERT).

In *Women and the Crisis in Sex Hormones,* Barbara Seaman and Gideon Seaman[54] compiled an impressive amount of evidence that reveals the harmful effects of sex hormones, such as the birth control pill, diethylstilbestrol (DES), and ERT. The studies showing a positive link between ERT users and a significant increase in incidence of endometrial cancer [cancer of the membrane lining the inner surface of the uterus][55] have been criticized for methodological reasons by some physicians. Thus, many physicians continue to prescribe ERT; they also fought against government attempts to place a warning on bottle labels. In January 1979, the *New England Journal of Medicine* published an article reporting the findings of a large case-control study headed by a group of researchers at Johns Hopkins University.[56] This carefully controlled study should put an end to the controversy. The researchers conclude unequivocally that ERT increases the risk of endometrial cancer.

> Our case-control study of the relation between estrogen use and endometrial cancer involved 451 cases and 888 controls. The overall risk of endometrial carcinoma [cancer] was sixfold for estrogen users as compared with non-users; long-term users (five years) had a 15-fold risk. Excess risk was present for both diethylstilbestrol and conjugated estrogens. The risk associated with cyclic use was as great as that for continuous use . . . This investigation contradicts the speculation that the association between this cancer and estrogen use can be explained by swifter diagnosis for estrogen users, misclassification of estrogen-related hyperplasia or treatment of early symptoms of the tumor with estrogen.[57]

Women who have had hysterectomies are obviously not at risk of endometrial cancer because the endometrium has been removed. However, the Seamans argue that ERT is not safe even for these women because the risk of breast cancer also increases with ERT use. Though fewer studies report a link between breast cancer and ERT, the Seamans quote research that also appeared in the *New England Journal of Medicine* and state:

> During the first five years of estrogen use, breast cancer does not increase. It may even occur less frequently than it does among women who are taking hormones. But after five years the risks start rising. Fifteen years after commencing therapy [twice as many ERT patients have] breast cancer as women who never used it. The length of time a woman stays on ERT does not seem to matter. What counts is simply the number of years that have passed since her first exposure. Dosages do matter, though, and the usual daily dose prescribed in the United States — 1.25 or 2.5 mg — is associated with breast cancer many years later. Women who have had benign breast diseases ordinarily face twice the usual risk of developing breast cancer later. If, however, the benign breast disease occurred after [they took] ERT, cancer risks increase sevenfold.[58]

Some hysterectomies are necessary and lifesaving* but one must conclude with the Seamans that it makes no sense to accept unnecessary surgery followed by an unnecessary and potentially dangerous drug.

There are other less life-threatening but disturbing side effects to the hysterectomy. Noting the limitations of available data and urging more long-term study, Niles Newton did an extensive review of the worldwide literature on hysterectomy and concluded that

> repeated or controlled studies indicate that hysterectomy may yield problems for some women in the following areas: rejection by male partners, hot flushes after con-

* See page 255 for the list, compiled by the Boston Women's Health Book Collective in *Our Bodies, Ourselves,* of indications that a hysterectomy is needed.

> servation of ovarian tissue, severe hot flushes after ovariectomy, long-term psychourinary problems, weight changes, lingering fatigue and prolonged convalescence, painful intercourse, depression, sleep disturbances and other psychiatric symptoms.[59]

There is also some reason to believe that the physical changes accomplished by the surgery may alter sexual response. Despite the importance of this question, most studies have focused on the psychological reactions to hysterectomy.[60] Though there is an absence of systematic empirical research on sexual response after a hysterectomy, gynecologists usually tell women that their sex lives will improve or that there will be no change. For example, "In the long term, far from hysterectomy marking a stage in the running down of sexual function, removal of the uterus should result in an increase in sexual activity and enjoyment."[61]

I am not suggesting that women become inorgasmic after a hysterectomy. Undoubtedly some women do experience increased sexual satisfaction after the correction of a painful or debilitating pelvic condition or after the fear of pregnancy has been removed. However, this does not prove that sexual response remains the same. Carefully considering Masters and Johnson's findings on the physiology of female sexuality, Susanne Morgan points out the types of changes that may affect sexual responses. Since the uterus is involved in each stage of female arousal, including excitement, plateau, orgasm, and resolution, there is the potential for a change in each stage when the uterus is absent. Morgan states:

> During the excitement phase, a general characteristic is a rush of blood to the entire pelvic area, called vasocongestion, which causes the feeling of arousal. If the uterus is not there, there is less tissue to become aroused. The uterus is elevated during the excitement phase, and the vagina balloons, increasing in diameter by as much as three times, and in length by as much as an inch . . .

> During the plateau phase there is further elevation and ballooning, and the uterus increases in size, becoming as much as twice its size. The extra increment of sexual tension will not be felt by a woman after hysterectomy. During orgasm, the uterus contracts, and the more severe the orgasm, the stronger the contraction, suggesting that after hysterectomy orgasms may not reach the intensity they may have before. In the resolution phase the sexual tension recedes, but in some women additional orgasms can follow, especially if she maintains plateau-level sexual tension. Since after hysterectomy there is less vasocongestion than with an intact uterus, it could be predicted that multiple orgasms would be less likely after a hysterectomy than before.[62]

Morgan also points out that if the ovaries have been removed and estrogen levels are low, there will be less or slower vaginal lubrication. This is significant because lubrication is the first indication of sexual tension for women, similar to erection in a male. Slower lubrication can cause the woman problems in interpreting sexual cues as well as pain on penile entry. The surgeon's repair of the vagina is also crucial. A penis striking a scarred area can result in painful intercourse. More research is obviously needed before gynecologists can truthfully tell women that sexual response is not affected by hysterectomy.

Considering all of the available evidence that indicates the hysterectomy involves a long operating time, significant morbidity, prolonged hospitalization, considerable blood loss, and a number of other physical and social side effects, one can only conclude that hysterectomy is unacceptable as a means of sterilization, especially since the tubal ligation accomplishes the same objective and is simpler, safer, and less expensive. The idea of a prophylactic hysterectomy may, in fact, be a contradiction in terms.

Notes

1. Russell C. Scott, *The World of a Gynecologist* (London: Oliver and Boyd, 1968), p. 25.
2. Eliot Freidson, *Profession of Medicine* (New York: Dodd, Mead and Company, 1973).
3. David Burkons and J. Robert Willson, "Is the Obstetrician-Gynecologist a Specialist or a Primary Physician to Women?" *American Journal of Obstetrics and Gynecology*, 121 (1975), 808.
4. Howard Taylor, "Objectives and Principles in the Training of the Obstetrician-Gynecologist: Training for Surgical Virtuosity and Versatility or for Public Service," *American Journal of Surgery* 110, (1965), 37.
5. Diana Scully and Pauline Bart, "A Funny Thing Happened on the Way to the Orifice: Women in Gynecology Texts," *American Journal of Sociology*, 78 (1973), 1045–1051.
6. Willard Cooke, *Essentials of Gynecology* (Philadelphia: J. B. Lippincott, 1943).
7. Ralph Benson, *Handbook of Obstetrics and Gynecology* (Los Altos, California: Lange Medical Publishers, 1971).
8. Cooke, *Essentials of Gynecology*, pp. 59–60.
9. Ibid., p. 60.
10. Emil Novak and Edmund R. Novak, *Textbook of Gynecology* (Baltimore: Williams and Wilkins Company, 1952), p. 572.
11. Alfred C. Kinsey, et al., *Sexual Behavior in the Human Female* (New York: Simon and Schuster, 1953).
12. Mary Jane Sherfey, *The Nature and Evolution of Female Sexuality* (New York: Random House, 1972).
13. I. C. Rubin and Josef Novak, *Integrated Gynecology: Principles and Practice*, Vol. III (New York: McGraw-Hill Book Company, 1956), p. 77.
14. Langdon Parsons and Sheldon C. Sommers, *Gynecology* (Philadelphia: W. B. Saunders Company, 1962), p. 494.
15. Ruth Brecher and Edward Brecher, *An Analysis of Human Sexual Response* (New York: New American Library, 1966).
16. Thomas Jeffcoate, *Principles of Gynecology* (London: Butterworth, 1967), p. 726.
17. Ibid.
18. Edmund R. Novak, Georgeanna Seegar Jones, and Howard Jones, Jr., *Novak's Textbook of Gynecology* (Baltimore: Williams and Wilkins Company, 1970), p. 662.
19. Brecher and Brecher, *An Analysis of Human Sexual Response*, p. 276.
20. Ibid.
21. Pauline Bart, "From Those Wonderful People That Brought You

the Vaginal Orgasm: Sex Education for Medical Students." Unpublished paper presented at the meetings of the American Sociological Association, 1976.
22. John Mudd and Richard Siegel, "Sexuality — The Experience and Anxieties of Medical Students," *New England Journal of Medicine,* 281 (1969), 1397–1403.
23. Ibid., p. 1402.
24. Bernard Kutner, "Surgeons and Their Patients: A Study in Social Perceptions," in *Patients, Physicians and Illness,* E. Gartly Jaco, ed. (Glencoe: The Free Press, 1958), p. 395.
25. Lilliam Runnerstrom, "The Effectiveness of Nurse-Midwifery in a Supervised Hospital Environment," *Bulletin of the American College of Nursing Midwives,* 14 (1968), 52.
26. Nancy Stoller Shaw, "'So You're Going to Have a Baby . . .' Institutional Processing of Maternity Patients." Ph.D. dissertation, Brandeis University, 1972. My observations did not include the nursery. However, Shaw states that care in the nursery was "horrifying." Nurses told her they had to keep washing the babies "not for cleanliness but to get the smell from the mothers off them." Other types of care were ignored, such as holding the baby while feeding.
27. Julius Roth, "Care of the Sick: Professionalism vs. Love." Paper presented at the Pacific Medical Center Symposium on the Medical Mystique, March, 1973.
28. John Bunker, "Surgical Manpower," *New England Journal of Medicine,* 282 (1970), 3.
29. Charles Lewis, "Variation in the Incidence of Surgery," *New England Journal of Medicine,* 281 (1969), 880–884.
30. Rita Nickerson, et al., "Doctors Who Perform Operations," *New England Journal of Medicine,* 295 (1976), 921–926.
31. Eugene G. McCarthy, "Second Opinion Surgical Program: A Vehicle for Cost Containment." Unpublished Report to the American Medical Association's Commission on the Cost of Medical Care, 1977.
32. Victor Cohn, "No. 1 Operation Now: Hysterectomy," Washington *Post,* May 10, 1977.
33. John Bunker, "Elective Hysterectomy: Pro and Con," *New England Journal of Medicine,* 295 (1976), 264–268.
34. McCarthy, "Second Opinion."
35. Frank Dyck, et al., "Effect of Surveillance on the Number of Hysterectomies in the Province of Saskatchewan," *New England Journal of Medicine,* 296 (1977), 1326–1328.
36. Joann Rodgers, "The Rush to Surgery," *New York Times Magazine,* September 21, 1975, p. 34.

37. Niles Newton, "Reactions to Hysterectomy: Fact or Fiction," *Primary Care*, 3 (1976), 781–801.
38. William W. Jack, Vergil Slee, and Peter Headly, "Gynecological Surgery: Its Profile," *American Journal of Obstetrics and Gynecology*, 89 (1964), 193.
39. Novak, Jones, and Jones, *Novak's Textbook*, 1970 edition, p. 271.
40. Lester T. Hibbard, "Sexual Sterilization by Elective Hysterectomy," *American Journal of Obstetrics and Gynecology*, 112 (1972), 1082.
41. Novak, Jones, and Jones, *Novak's Textbook*, 1970 edition, p. 94.
42. Ibid., 1975 edition, p. 112.
43. Ibid., p. 112.
44. Ibid., p. 113.
45. Ibid.
46. J. B. Skelton, "Prophylactic Hysterectomy and Salpingo-Oophorectomy — Is It or Is It Not Good Preventive Medicine," *Audio Digest of Obstetrics and Gynecology*, 20 (1973).
47. *New York Times*, February 1, 1976.
48. See William Ledger and Margaret Child, "The Hospital Care of Patients Undergoing Hysterectomy: An Analysis of 12,026 Patients from the Professional Activity Study," *American Journal of Obstetrics and Gynecology*, 117 (1973); also Russell K. Laros and Bruce A. Work, "Female Sterilization," *American Journal of Obstetrics and Gynecology*, 122 (1975); also Hibbard, "Sexual Sterilization."
49. Hibbard, "Sexual Sterilization," p. 1082.
50. Laros and Work, "Female Sterilization," p. 697.
51. Bernard Rosenfeld, Sidney Wolfe, and Robert McGarrah, "Study of Surgical Sterilization: Present Abuses and Proposed Regulations" (Washington, D.C., Health Research Group, October 1973), p. 2.
52. Victor Cohn, "U.S. Moves to Curb Unneeded Surgery," Washington *Post*, November 2, 1977.
53. Rosenfeld, et al., "Study of Surgical Sterilization," p. 2.
54. Barbara Seaman and Gideon Seaman, *Women and the Crisis in Sex Hormones* (New York: Rawson Associates, 1977).
55. See Thomas M. Mack, "Estrogens and Endometrial Cancer in a Retirement Community," *New England Journal of Medicine*, 284 (1976), 1262–1267.
56. Carlos Antunes, Paul Stolley, Neil Rosenshein, Joan Davies, Janes Tonascia, Charles Brown, Lonnie Burnett, Ann Rutledge, Merle Pokempner, and Rafael García, "Endometrial Cancer and Estrogen Use," *New England Journal of Medicine*, 300 (1979), 9–13.
57. Antunes et al., "Endometrial Cancer," p. 9.
58. Seaman and Seaman, *Women and the Crisis in Sex Hormones*, p. 338.
59. Newton, "Reactions to Hysterectomy," p. 799.

60. Janet Polivy, "Psychological Reactions to Hysterectomy: A Critical Review," *American Journal of Obstetrics and Gynecology,* 118 (1974), 417–426.
61. A. G. Amias, "Sexual Life After Gynaecological Operations — I," *British Medical Journal* (June 1975), 608–609.
62. Susanne Morgan, "Sexuality After Hysterectomy and Castration," *Women and Health,* 3 (1978), 5–10.

V

Learning to Be a Surgeon

NEWLY GRADUATED PHYSICIANS elect to enter a residency program because it is the way for them to acquire additional training and secure the opportunity to develop the skills of their profession. During their years in medical school, students receive a general grounding in medicine by studying the basic sciences and observing various clinical situations. Students are also allowed to perform certain routine tasks, usually the work others with more advanced training don't want to do, such as taking histories, starting IVs, drawing blood for tests, and performing uncomplicated examinations. In this way, some actual experience in medical work is acquired. At Elite and Mass, medical students were permitted to perform on institutional patients such simple tasks as a dilation and curettage or a spontaneous vaginal delivery, and sometimes they were allowed to assist at a more complex procedure, like a tubal ligation.

Because of the time needed to acquire a general grounding in medical knowledge and because of the relatively brief exposure to each specialty area, newly graduated doctors lack experience. Medical students frequently spoke of their difficulty with basic obstetrical and gynecological technique. Ovaries, for example, are not easy for an untrained hand to locate. Typically, a medical student who excitedly explained that he had just examined a sixteen-week-size uterine fibroid and could really feel the tumor told me, "To tell you the truth, most of the time when they [attendings or residents] ask me to examine a patient, I can't feel anything. To be honest, I'm not sure that I have ever really felt ovaries." (Field Notes, Elite.) Similarly, a third-year resident at Mass explained that when he began his residency and did a pelvic examination, he couldn't feel anything. Now, he said, he can really distinguish between a normal pelvis and one with a problem. (Interview, Mass.)

First-year residents who had completed an internship had a slight advantage over those who had not. But though they were more familiar with medicine in general, they still lacked experience in the specific skills required of an obstetrician-gynecologist. Take this description of a tubal ligation performed by an intern assisted by a fourth-year resident:

> He was very clumsy, his hands shook, he dropped instruments, instruments opened up when they shouldn't, he had to be told from what end to begin stitching. At one point he dropped an instrument into the incision and couldn't retrieve it. He started to touch an organ and the resident yelled not to grab anything until he was sure what it was — it could be a bowel. He appeared to be doing everything wrong. When it was over he thanked the resident, who, with relief in his voice, simply said, "Nice job." (Field Notes, Elite.)

"Practicing" Medicine

The years spent in an ACOG board–certified residency program are intended to transform the neophyte into a highly skilled physician. Training programs expose residents to patients who present problems of various types and orders of complexity. Through playing the role of specialist for these patients, residents were expected to perfect their obstetrical and gynecological techniques.

Though the tenet is not exclusive to surgery, it is especially true that when the skills to be acquired are surgical, learning is believed to be possible only through doing. Textbooks, it is thought, cannot teach one how or when to remove a uterus, nor do they adequately describe pathology in all its variety and detail. Residents frequently told me that their patients were not the same as textbook cases.

Surgical skill was acquired primarily through repetition and practice. Since it was believed that increased exposure would result, up to a point, in increased expertise, a resident was obliged to practice a skill or technique until he thought he had mastered it, or, more accurately, until he was confident enough of his ability to perform it without assistance.

Because the residents were hired by the institution, in part, to acquire skills and judgment, emphasis was placed not on how competent they were in performing a certain skill, but rather on how technically incompetent they were. Lack of expertise was acceptable unless a resident was considered indifferent about learning or exhibited a level of skill below what might be reasonably expected at his level of training. In general, lack of expertise in residency was interpreted to mean the resident was in need of more practice.

Attendings sometimes reminded residents of their obligation to practice. For example, during a lecture on the application of forceps, residents were told that they didn't take enough advantage of the opportunity to apply forceps. The attending explained that when he was a resident, he tried to give every woman in labor a cervical block and a forceps delivery until he had mastered the technique. (Field Notes, Elite.) Similarly, a resident advised a medical student what to do with a woman about to deliver twins: "The best thing you can do if you have never delivered twins is to deliver them yourself. Of course, this may not be the best thing for the patient." (Field Notes, Mass.)

In return for the opportunity to acquire advanced training, residents agree to perform a service for the hospital. In a facility like Elite, residents also agree to offer a service to the attending staff by assisting them in the care of their private patients, with the expectation that they would be rewarded by being allowed to do a certain amount of the attendings' private surgery. In training institutions such as Elite and Mass, residents provide patient services at a salary considerably less than what they would receive in a private setting. From the resident's perspective, however, the main function of a residency was not to provide patient care but to gain training.

> I don't look at residency as a job, which unfortunately I think the hospital does. We talked about this before — how much of it is education, how much patient care, how much of it is doing things for other doctors. As far as I am concerned, my only responsibility or my major responsibility is to get my education at this point, and my responsibility for providing patient care for the hospital or community is really quite negligible as far as I am concerned, but I have to give that in order to get my education. (Interview, Elite.)

> I recognize that during a residency you do provide service to a community that needs service, but I think that the prime goal and the most important feature of a training program is to train. (Interview, Elite.)

Some residents de-emphasized their responsibility to provide patient care because they felt unqualified. One especially sensitive resident explained:

> As I see it, a resident is here to work and to learn. He should be learning on the private patients as much as on the institutional patients. I don't feel that I am in the position to be offering first-class medical care to anybody. I'm not qualified; that's the way I look at it. If anybody expects us to be the doctor for these patients, they are asking for second-class medical care. (Interview, Elite.)

Residents even made a cognitive distinction between "practicing" medicine while in training and the "practice" of medicine. The resident saw himself as "practicing" skills in order to become proficient before embarking upon the "practice" of medicine as a highly skilled specialist.

In discussing their professional identification, only residents about to complete their training spoke of themselves as obstetrician-gynecologists. A resident's main identity during training was that of someone in the process of becoming trained; his major preoccupation was gettting as much as possible out of the residency.

The basic dilemma in providing health care to institutional patients, who are usually the poor or minority-group members, is that residents are expected to deliver medical services they are not yet trained to provide. People who receive health care under such conditions thereby become "teaching material" for a physician-in-training who has not yet mastered the skill he is practicing. Put another way, the poor are expected to be satisfied with receiving their health care from the least qualified rather than the most qualified physician, a situation the more affluent members of society would hardly tolerate.

• • •

In general, the work from which residents derived the greatest satisfaction — and the experience residents sought out — was that which they believed would contribute most to their learning and development. But skills can't be practiced unless patients are available who present medical problems fitting a resident's training needs. Consequently, the most important resource in training were patients who had illnesses with the potential for increasing the resident's knowledge and skill. The patients' needs were a secondary consideration.

> A D & C in residency, I don't like to do. Certain patients need these D & Cs . . . but I don't like to do them because it is a pain in the neck. A patient with dysfunctional bleeding needs a D & C, but I don't get anything out of it. It's just a lot of paper work to do a five-minute operation. As a private practitioner it's a whole different thing. There is a financial aspect to it and there may be more obligation

> to patients that need to have it. I don't feel this with certain patients over here. (Interview, Elite.)

At both Elite and Mass, some work was regarded with nearly universal dislike and was usually referred to as "dirty work" or "scut work." Described by one first-year resident, scut work included "drawing blood, starting IVs, filling out forms, paper work, nursing care, going with patients to pelvimetry, chasing after x-ray reports, calling up labs — things that nurses, technicians, or aides should be doing." (Interview, Elite.) A redeeming virtue could be found in this type of work only if the resident felt he had lacked the opportunity to do it in medical school. For example, a first-year resident remarked:

> One gets to the point where you get tired of drawing blood for cross and type match and of starting IVs. But to me, because I didn't do an internship, I probably don't despise it as much as one who had . . . I strongly disliked it by the end of the year because I thought I had enough, but initially, starting out, I was sort of glad to have it. (Interview, Elite.)

Because of what residents referred to as the "dumping syndrome," junior residents were often required to do undesirable work. As one fourth-year resident at Elite put it, "Dirty work rolls down." In answer to the question "How are the duties of a first-year resident defined," at Elite I would frequently be told, "It is to do whatever the second-, third-, and fourth-year residents and attending don't want to do."

Surgical skills were acquired gradually through apprenticeship. This meant that junior residents were expected to begin training by performing simple tasks and, as exposure increased and as basic skills were acquired, move on to more difficult procedures. At Elite, the structure of the services reflected the apprenticeship format, and various levels of training were combined on each service. Under this system, senior residents occupied positions that carried the greatest privilege. One important advantage was that they had relatively greater freedom of choice over the work they did. At Mass, before changes in the program, members of each service were closer to the same level of training, so rank, status, and privilege tended to blur. Under these conditions, undesirable work was more likely to be shared by members of a service instead of being passed down the hierarchical ladder.

At Elite, the dumping syndrome was exaggerated by another factor. It was the stated position of the department that medical students rotating through Elite for training in obstetrics and gynecology should not be required to do dirty work. The Chair, who was dedicated to raising the caliber of medical students choosing to specialize in obstetrics and gynecology, believed that one way to attract medical students to his program when they chose their residencies was to make the time they spent there during medical school as pleasant and rewarding as possible. Therefore, medical students could not be required to run errands, start IVs, and the like. They did such tasks only if they wanted to. In April, the Chair was pleased because two "very good" medical students who had been exposed to this special treatment chose to enter the residency. However, when these students started to do the work of first-year residents, they were surprised to find that they had "got to do more as students than they did as residents." This does not mean that first-year residents didn't actually work, but, rather, that they did not consider most of the work they did a learning experience.

Elite also lacked interns on whom to dump unwanted work. The hierarchical structure combined with the lack of assistance from medical students and interns created a situation in which first-year residents were forced to perform a considerable amount of scut work, as well as those tasks their seniors no longer wanted to do and were in a position to avoid. At Elite, the service that most clearly exemplified the problem for first-year residents was private gynecology:

> First of all, you have patients to make rounds on every morning and they are private patients and they don't want

> to see you anyway. That's a great way to start the day. That has to be done before surgery is started at 7:45 A.M. Then you had to get scrubbed and ready for surgery and you weren't going to do it [surgery].
>
> I ended up with the worst cases of all. I spent many Tuesdays and Thursdays doing nothing but peritoneoscopies, during which time I would do nothing but hold the uterus on a stick. I think a certain amount of that is necessary; you have to know what is going on before you can be expected to do anything. I did some minor things. They would always turn over a D & C to you but by that time I had done plenty of D & Cs, and they were no good anyway. Not that I couldn't learn anything from them, but you know, it's no big thrill to do a D & C. There were a few minor things that I got to do. They let you close the abdomen, but I did that as a medical student so I wasn't too thrilled about that either. To me it was a considerable amount of work for very little gain. (Interview, Elite.)

A resident who came to Elite with more experience than the average resident expressed it this way:

> Private gyn was a waste of time. I did a lot of work with no return. They say you get a return in your third year because in your third year you start doing all the cases, but you really are a peon. It was hard for me because for three years I was on my own and for three years I have always had at least ten people working for me to do all this junk. (Interview, Elite.)

The objective of first-year residents at Elite became, as one resident put it, "trying to do more technically, trying to learn more, and trying to do as little of the actual dirty work as possible." (Interview, Elite.)

Another almost universally disliked aspect of the resident's work was the time spent in the clinics. After spending several months observing at Elite and Mass, I realized that the foremost skill required of residents was speed. In fact, there was a marked difference in the amount of time it took for a new resident, as opposed to a seasoned resident, to complete an examination. "Slow" residents were reminded that there were fifty more patients waiting.

At Mass, where residents in general had greater patient awareness, some residents disliked the clinics because of the quality of care they were forced to give there.

> The clinic is just overburdened. It's ridiculous to assign two ob residents to the morning ob clinic when you have anywhere from 100 to 150 patients to see in three hours. About all you can do is shake hands and say good-bye. Each resident has to see about 50 patients in three hours, and that's no way to give health care.
>
> We are always afraid that we are going to miss something because we have to go so fast. And if you don't [see all of the ob patients], there is another problem. The gyn clinic follows right after and they have to clear that area. (Interview, Mass.)

In contrast to this, at Elite dislike for the clinic was often related to a distaste for the patients treated there as much as to the nature of the work.

> I just . . . I'm bored with the clinic. I couldn't relate well with patients. I didn't feel that the patients understood what I was saying, and sometimes I didn't understand what the patients were saying. To me it is just very boring and tedious; seeing 50 or 60 patients a day is just craziness. (Interview, Elite.)

> I did a rotation in the clinic, which is a pain in the ass and requires a lot of screening, prenatal care, treating the masses, providing a service for the hospital. (Interview, Elite.)

Although residents in both programs disliked clinic work because it was "boring and routine," there were more complaints at Elite, where, for ten weeks each year, residents did nothing but see patients in the clinic, which meant they were not scheduled to do surgery. At Mass, on the other hand, clinic service was integrated with obstetrics and surgery. On a typical day a resident might spend the morning in surgery and the afternoon in the gynecology clinic. Under this arrangement, the clinic could be used to the resident's advantage.

> You have to understand, as I see it, the clinic is our source of patients. You know, the Pap smear clinic; you see about 70 percent of the patients with PID and vaginal discharge and these routine things. But many times you get a hysterectomy. (Interview, Elite.)

At Mass, pathology discovered in the clinics could be utilized to advance the resident's own professional knowledge and development. That is, residents in the gynecology division used the clinics to find surgical cases they could treat. At Elite, however, "nice cases" found in the clinic had to be turned over to the chief of the ward gynecology service. Thus, because residents didn't receive a return on their clinic work, they found it to be an unrewarding experience.

> It was just scut work for a second-year resident on the clinic rotation. What I would be seeing was postop sections, postop hysterectomies, patients with abnormal Pap smears. Nothing to do with them, no responsibility whatsoever. If something came up and I found a patient that I thought needed surgery, I just got the chief from ward gyn service and said, "I think I have a case for you; here it is," and go on to the next one. (Interview, Elite.)

A resident's attitude about those aspects of his work originally regarded with disfavor could undergo subtle change if his doing that work was reinterpreted as contributing significantly to his professional development. This seemed to be the case with oncology at Mass.

Initially, residents in both programs expressed an aversion to "sick" or terminally ill patients. Avoidance of terminal illness had been a factor in their choice of obstetrics and gynecology as a specialty. Oncology patients were certainly among the sickest of patients. At Mass, however, which had a training program for specialists in oncology (referred to by residents as "radical surgery"), some residents underwent subtle attitude changes with regard to dying patients once they understood the benefit they could derive from experience in oncologic surgery. Residents who had mastered regular surgery to their own satisfaction were attracted to oncology as a means to improve their surgical technique and operative speed. One Mass resident who at first was uninterested in oncology said that his opinion started to change during his third year of residency.

> I was attracted to it to improve my surgical technique and I wanted to get a chance to do some of the surgeries that we don't get a chance to do otherwise . . . When it comes to practice, I may do regular gyn surgery for the rest of my life, but when it comes to training, I found that there was nothing else that I could improve upon in regular surgery.
>
> So if you go for radical surgery, you get more experience and gradually you find other things easier to do. You get more competent. In regular surgery, you try to avoid touching other areas; you just take the uterus. In radical surgery, you dissect out everything; you look for everything. That way, you expose yourself to more danger, that way you know more, you are better oriented to the pelvis. So it gives you better in-depth orientation surgerywise. (Interview, Mass.)

Another Mass senior resident expressed it this way:

> I do enjoy it, and I think any doctor is lucky to do radical surgery. I was lucky enough to do seven or eight and after that, you know that minor surgery is just a simple thing.

> A hysterectomy — at first you do it in three or four hours. But after you do a radical, you can do it in one hour. You get more oriented in radical surgery. (Interview, Mass.)

Using a number of techniques to avoid unwanted tasks,[1] the major preoccupation of residents, at all levels of training, was securing "meaningful" work, which usually meant some form of surgery. This need was so deeply experienced that residents would say they were "hungry for surgery," when, for some reason, they had difficulty locating cases.

> In the beginning, it [surgery] was a challenge . . . and I wanted to have more because that is why I came here. Because to be hungry all the time for surgery, it's very bad. (Interview, Elite.)

Obstetrics and gynecology is a field in which most of the work can be described as routine, preventive, or well care.[2] Residents estimated that as much as 90 percent of private practice consisted of this type of medical care. In other words, the largest slice of an obstetrician-gynecologist's time is spent doing Pap smears, dispensing birth control information, treating vaginal infections, and providing prenatal well care — exactly the same work, only more profitable and pleasant in private practice, that residents considered a waste of time in training and found so boring in the clinics. During residency, they were interested in pathology, and surgery was regarded as the most desirable aspect of their job.

> You are interested in pathology . . . because you never know when a woman is going to have a normal vaginal delivery until the moment that this happens. But what I am interested in is the abnormality . . . seeing pathology. But in order to detect the abnormal, you have to follow the normal ones. There are patients who are really high-risk patients and this is what you are interested in. Let's say you have a diabetic, a patient with a history of still-

> borns, it's the pathology you are interested in. (Interview, Mass.)

An interesting or rare case aroused general interest among the residents, who attempted to learn as much as possible from it.

> When you have an interesting patient, you get as much out of the patient as possible regarding the disease the patient has. If I have a patient with sickle cell anemia, then I should learn as much as possible about that disease. (Interview, Mass.)

Ironically, the type of care that would occupy the majority of private practice was considered least important in training, where residents learned to place the greatest value on work involving surgery.

Mastery of Skills

Although the overwhelming emphasis in training was on doing surgery, residents did not expect nor did they want to do an unlimited amount of surgery. On the contrary, residents had a specific idea of how much experience they needed with each procedure. An advanced resident explained:

> I would like to do more vaginal surgery, more surgery for stress incontinence. I feel I can do it, but I would like to do more. Doing ten or twenty is OK, but it is better if you can say that you did more than twenty of each procedure. I got to do only two surgeries for stress incontinence, which means that I can't approach every case with the same skill. (Interview, Mass.)

A junior resident explained what he needed in obstetrics:

> I do feel confident. The only thing that I think I need experience in is surgical cases, such as cesarean sections.

> So far I have done fifteen. That's a good number to start with, to feel confident, but now you have to perfect your own technique. You have to go through cases, especially repeat cesarean sections. From below [vaginally], I think I have enough, though probably I need some more twin deliveries. I have done four or five but you need fifteen or twenty. At least you have to do some. (Interview, Mass.)

In general, the number of cases that residents hoped to secure for each type of surgery varied according to the difficulty or rarity of the procedure, the amount of time spent on the service where the skill was practiced, the profession's and department's emphases, and, also important, on a reasonable expectation of the amount of pathology obtainable.

From the residents' point of view there was a problem because "material" is not distributed according to the skills they needed to practice. For example, a patient requiring dilation and curettage is easier to find than a patient needing an abdominal hysterectomy. Spontaneous vaginal deliveries are more common than cesarean sections, and both are more frequent than cesarean hysterectomies. Thus, the opportunity to practice some skills was more easily obtained because the problems that demanded them were more abundant in the patient population. Other skills, corresponding to rarer pathology, were much more difficult to practice because the opportunities presented themselves less often. Because surgical training was progressive in the sense that rarer or more difficult cases were reserved for senior years, residents experienced increased difficulty locating pathology appropriate to their training needs.

The value of the work done during training varied in relation to how the resident assessed his deficiencies and needs. As a result, the type of work he sought depended on his level of training and the amount of experience he had accumulated at that time. A forceps delivery, prized in the first year, was generally avoided by the third year, when the resident became satisfied with the amount of experience he had had with the procedure. Similarly, a junior resident did not expect to have the opportunity to do vaginal, cesarean, or postpartum hysterectomies, which, because of their rarity or complexity, were reserved for senior residents.

Every resident kept a record of the number of each procedure he performed and was aware at any point of what he lacked in experience. As a result, he could state exactly the types of cases for which he was looking. During the second-year rotation in obstetrics at Elite, for instance, a resident was no longer interested in doing spontaneous vaginal deliveries. He wanted to perform more complicated techniques, like forceps rotations.

> In the second year you know exactly what you are looking for and you see who is doing the right job. You know exactly what technique is better than the other. You are trying to do more specific things, like rotation forceps. (Interview, Elite.)

The same situation existed at every level of training. For example, during his senior years, a resident was chiefly interested in mastering gynecological surgery.

> I need more hysterectomies, vaginal and abdominal . . . I need to sharpen up a little bit on hysterectomies. So far I haven't done enough, I think. I thought I would never have enough sections, but eventually I said I had enough. And again, more complications. I have to see an injured bowel, an injured bladder, I haven't been involved with that yet.
>
> [Q. Because you haven't injured any yet?]
>
> Right, because I haven't done enough yet. Eventually I will do it and then I will feel confident. (Interview, Elite.)

The need to do surgery was temporal. When a surgical procedure that once was sought because of its learning value was mastered, it decreased in value to the resident.

> Yes, I was really content by the end. I really didn't have to be greedy about them [cesarean sections]. I could pass

> them on. I didn't have to grab all the time, I was so satisfied. (Interview, Mass.)

In general, once a procedure or technique was mastered, or the resident believed he had mastered it, he would cease to perform it. If possible, he would avoid patients with the corresponding problem or pathology, often by dumping or by giving them to residents still in need of practice. A fourth-year resident explained:

> I'm not looking for surgery that much anymore. Once you get to know how to do it and you are satisfied that you can do it, then you stop looking for it usually. (Interview, Mass.)

This surgical hiatus was situational and should not be interpreted to mean that the resident had tired of performing the procedure or that he would always avoid such surgery. Rather, it meant that while he was in training, the resident was interested mostly in practicing what he had not yet mastered.

> After you do seventy or eighty normal deliveries, you don't want to do them anymore. It isn't that you don't like to do them, but you are more interested in doing complicated cases and in seeing as much pathology as you can. (Interview, Mass.)

Thus, the type of experience a resident sought during his training was related to a composite of the experiences that had preceded it. As a resident became skilled, his point of reference changed, as did his attitude toward his work. One resident put it this way:

> As a student, you like the bizarre things. "I saw it," you say to everybody. As an intern you try to learn how to handle things. As a resident you want more experience. As an attending you want the easiest and simplest things,

> so it really changes. And during the years of residency it changes also. For example, I know in the first year, I wanted to do as many forceps as possible, and this is just because of the selfish idea that I need the training. In case I need it; everything is in case I need it. Part of being a doctor is the buildup of a very tough layer of skin, very thick layer of confidence in yourself. (Interview, Elite.)

Because the resident was doing work that he had not as yet mastered, the concept of error took on a special meaning in training. A resident was expected to make errors. A fourth-year resident explained:

> It is by making mistakes that you grow and mature as a physician. You learn not to do it again; I think that is important. Because if I wasn't ever going to make any mistakes, there wouldn't be any reason for me to spend four years being a resident. (Interview, Elite.)

Although errors frequently met with oral censure, sometimes severe and humiliating from the attending staff, if the resident was able to attribute the problem to a reasonable lack of experience, he could also relieve somewhat his feeling of responsibility for the act.

> The errors that are made, well, very few of them are errors of indifference or neglect or anything like that. It's just a case of not knowing, and I think that if there is an error, that is a very valid excuse. I think that is why most of the errors are made. (Interview, Mass.)

Especially when supervision and teaching were minimal, the resident tended to perceive his errors as the unavoidable result of inexperience.

> I don't know if you can call it a mistake or something that you aren't experienced with and do something wrong.

> You can't call that a mistake. It's inexperience. If you aren't taught something, you can't do it. (Interview, Mass.)

On the other hand, when the error was due to a lack of knowledge or ability the resident believed he should have possessed, personal responsibility was more likely to be taken. A fourth-year resident said:

> Well, I think I have failed when I think I have done something wrong, something I should have known better. I can do something and it might not turn out right. But if I feel that I have done everything possible intellectually and technically to reach an end result that I think should be right — when I know my judgment may have been poor or that I am inadequate in a certain technical skill, where I should have had this technical skill, or I should have read about it, that's when I consider that I have really failed. (Interview, Elite.)

The lack of a concept of error in training is not confined to Elite and Mass. In their research on medical training in psychiatry and internal medicine, Stelling and Bucher also found that words such as "failure" and "mistake" didn't fit into the residents' vocabulary except in the case of wrong behavior, when "any well-trained person ought to know better."[3]

Developing Confidence

The resident's efforts toward gaining personal experience in a broad range of obstetrical and gynecological pathology while in training was related to the development of confidence in his professional ability. But determining exactly what confidence meant to the residents, or how confidence could be measured, was difficult because of the vagueness with which they applied the concept to themselves. A fourth-year resident attempted to explain confidence:

> I get the feeling now that I am as well trained as probably anyone else is in the country and in fact better trained in certain aspects . . . You go around and talk to people and every time you talk to someone new, they always bring up a case and they discuss their approach and you discuss your approach and you kind of know right from wrong — at least at this point of training — and you see how others approach it and you just feel that you are more confident in your approach and yours is the better approach. (Interview, Elite.)

Among other factors, confidence was related to the reduction of uncertainty. Sociologist Renée Fox[4] points out that despite scientific advances, the lives of modern physicians are still full of uncertainty. They must cope with their own imperfect or incomplete mastery of available knowledge and also must become reconciled to the fact that medical science is limited and cannot provide answers to every question. Fox found that medical students couldn't distinguish between these two types of uncertainty, which gave rise to an additional source of self-doubt. In contrast to medical students, residents were able to discriminate between "personal ignorance or ineptitude" and the "limitations of medical knowledge." Though little could be done about the latter, the elimination of personal deficiencies was thought possible, especially within the narrow limits of obstetrics and gynecology. Part of the appeal of the specialty is that it requires expertise in a relatively confined anatomical region of one sex. Significantly, residents believed it was possible to master obstetrics and gynecology in a way not possible in general surgery. At the same time, their confidence was threatened by the idea that a rare case may exist they hadn't yet seen.

> I don't think any resident in ob-gyn has had more opportunity to do things than I have. But there is always something that we have never done, you know, like the case now, the patient bleeding. No matter how old you are,

> you may be the oldest obstetrician in the hospital, and you may not have seen anything like that. There is always something you have never seen before. (Interview, Elite.)

As long as something remained unseen, the residents believed there was a problem they might not be able to handle. Lessening the gap between possible pathology and actual experience — that is, decreasing uncertainty — was a central concern of residents.

Because of the emphasis on pathology, programs in hospitals that have an institutional patient population are preferred by many residents over those that have only private patients. In the former situation, not only does the resident have his own patients on whom to practice, but poor people in general have poor health and present to the curious resident a greater amount and diversity of complications and pathology than do private patients.

> Even before I entered residency, I knew that a person like me wants more of the institutional patients, all the complications I can see. I realized that I wouldn't be so confident if I went through that residency in a suburban hospital; I wouldn't see complications. (Interview, Mass.)

Although they acknowledged the impossibility of experiencing every medical problem, residents expressed a sense of reduced uncertainty when they realized they were able to handle expertly and successfully the majority of obstetrical and gynecological problems without the assistance of a more experienced colleague.

> I would be writing, "Such and such needs to be done and Dr. So-and-So agrees, who called Dr. So-and-So." That's how it was in the beginning. But as I went on, I just said, "The patient needs this." I didn't write down So-and-So notified. I said, "I know what I am doing; I don't have to do that anymore." (Interview, Elite.)

Confidence also increased as the probability of confronting an unexpected problem or outcome was reduced. The less the subjective feeling of uncertainty in a situation, the greater the sense of confidence. For example, in response to my question "How confident do you feel?" one resident replied:

> It is hard to describe but you walk up on the labor row and you know that there are very few things that you aren't going to be able to handle, whereas when you walk up there the first day you think, I'm not going to be able to handle anything. (Interview, Mass.)

Another resident explained confidence this way:

> The first time you go to gyn, you don't feel confident and even if you read in the books, you don't find the same things in the books . . . especially here; they are different cases. You are scared. Sometimes when you are on call at night and have to cover the whole house for ob-gyn you think, If something happens, what am I going to do. Now I think if something happens, I can handle it . . . Confidence is like a foreign language; it comes slowly . . . To feel 100 percent confident is difficult. All the time you have your own questions. It is difficult to be perfect. (Interview, Mass.)

As the residents expressed it, when a surgeon walks into an operating room or delivery suite, he must feel in command of the situation, self-assured in his ability to anticipate and handle quickly whatever problems may unexpectedly occur. Stress is increased by a belief in the life-and-death nature of the surgical situation and was perhaps even more marked in childbirth, where, as I was frequently reminded, the lives of two patients were at stake. Because of these beliefs, confidence was considered an extremely important quality in surgeons, as is evident from the following remark made by an attending:

> My wife criticizes me because she says I think I know everything and always feel my way is best. I do have to feel that I know it all and that I can handle everything or else I can't do anything because I lack self-assurance. The same is true of residents. They must acquire this self-confidence in order to function. (Field Notes, Elite.)

Interestingly, we tend to think of confidence in terms of the patient's response to the physician. In order to maximize the benefits of a therapeutic relationship, it has been argued, the patient must trust and have confidence in the physician, who reciprocates by a responsible display of authority. Presumably, then, a self-assured, confident, authoritative presentation of self is intended to encourage and maintain the patient's confidence in the physician's ability. The research for this book, however, suggests that outward manifestations of confidence and self-assurance compose a core need for the surgeon himself. In fact, it is basic to his ability to function at all.

The resident's gradual accumulation of confidence in his ability to function autonomously was linked to his accepting responsibility for acts and decisions and was also related to the amount of supervision he needed or was given during the training process. Attending staff and residents alike believed that the residents' confidence could best be encouraged if they were not watched too closely. A first-year resident remarked:

> I would have preferred to see a little more supervision in spots, but I think that it turns out that because you didn't get that supervision, it helps you get off that crutch, stand up, be independent and assume the responsibility, instead of knowing that you can always rely on the crutch. (Interview, Elite.)

Initially, however, most of the residents at both Elite and Mass reported some apprehension and anxiety about their new roles. This was related to the fear that they might be called on to handle a problem for which they were technically unprepared. A resident who had just completed his first year at Elite said:

> I feel that I have more confidence in what is going on in the profession and I think that plays a key part because most of the first-year residents are very apprehensive and anxious about their roles as residents. They are afraid they may be called on to do something that they aren't really familiar with or haven't been trained in, and that is to be expected. So I think this year you feel much more confident about doing things and you aren't apprehensive in the middle of the night — "Oh, my God, what is it now!" (Interview, Elite.)

The amount and type of supervision at Elite and Mass was measurably different, and predictably this resulted in different experiences for the two sets of residents and their patients.

At Elite, residents were initially exposed to considerably more supervision than their peers at Mass. Most of it was by the senior resident on their service. Because the services were hierarchical, newcomers were provided with a role model, teacher, and supervisor. Elite residents could also take advantage of informal interaction with attendings, who, because their patients were treated in the same facility, were frequently present at the hospital. After an initial trial period, supervision was relaxed somewhat, and residents were expected to ask for help when they needed it. It was thus left to the individual to decide what he was capable of doing on his own.

> When you start off you get a lot of supervision; you don't know what you are doing. But as you get on and get the hang of the routine things, you get little supervision. Most of the time, the biggest part of medical education is knowing your limitations and seeking help when there is a problem. First you have to recognize a problem, then seek out an answer to it. You don't want to make decisions and

> take responsibility for things you aren't qualified for. (Interview, Elite.)

The program was designed to broaden gradually the range of responsibility residents were allowed or expected to assume. The result was that residents were allowed to get used to the program at a pace comfortable for them. Minor acts and decisions in labor and delivery could be carried out independently, but assistance could also be obtained if necessary.

The first structured opportunity to exercise independent action occurred in the second year, during the night shift in the labor and delivery rooms. Unlike the day shift, when the chief was on duty, at night the second-year resident was the most senior person present, and no one more experienced was immediately available to make difficult decisions. One resident related his experiences as follows:

> Nights were different. When you are the second-year resident at nights in the labor rooms, you have a lot more responsibility because there was no chief standing around all the time. You had to decide if there was a problem, and if there was, whether somebody senior to you should be notified. I found that I took a lot more responsibility on myself, almost as much as the chief would. (Interview, Elite.)

If the resident lacked the confidence to proceed on his own, he could call on senior people who were usually available. Some problems, such as emergency surgery, would almost always necessitate consultation and assistance. In general, though, the resident had some latitude and could work independently if he wanted to. The number and type of problems that he could handle without calling for help became the resident's gauge of his own, as well as others' ability and progress.

The third year of residency at Elite differed significantly from the first two. It was during this year that the resident became chief of the service in the clinic, the labor and delivery rooms, and in private gynecology. By far his most taxing yet satisfying experience in the third year was acting as chief of obstetrics. Rather than being supervised, the chief became the supervisor. Further, he was in the position to make decisions, exercise judgment, and take full responsibility for institutional patients. As one resident put it, "You know the buck stops with you, or at least if you choose to, you can have it stop with you." (Interview, Elite.) To the residents, the critical test was whether they were able to accept responsibility for their own acts and decisions. This experience prepared them for the challenge of their final year.

From the Elite resident's perspective, the most important experience of the fourth year, and perhaps of the entire residency, was the period he spent as chief of the ward gynecology service. Most significant to the residents, there was almost no supervision from attendings, so nearly full responsibility for institutional patients was placed on the chief. If help was needed, residents were expected to request it. A fourth-year resident explained:

> There are times that you may ask somebody for advice or help, but basically you are left pretty much to make your own decisions. On the gynecology service they [attendings] are supposed to examine all patients postoperatively. Our department, different from the surgical department, allows the chief resident to scrub on his own cases, without having an attending present. So pretty much you are in charge. (Interview, Elite.)

The ability to handle the role of chief became for the resident the final test of ability. One resident explained:

> The fourth year, the high point, the acme, the pinnacle of the whole program were those six months that you're chief, if you are able to stand on your own two feet, take a patient to the operating room, cut open an abdomen

> without anyone looking over your shoulder, telling you what to do . . . The six months that you are on ward gyn service are really valuable because that is the first chance you have to really stand on your own two feet and find out what it is all about, and if you are capable and prepared to assume all responsibility, you are generally allowed to. And we were and we could and we did. (Interview, Elite.)

Most important to the fourth-year resident was whether he had the confidence to assume responsibility for independent acts and decisions. The ability to handle the situation with confidence was crucial to a positive self-image and was used as a yardstick to measure his readiness to depart from the relatively protected training environment.

> I think that I learned an immense amount, and I think most of all I gained a lot of confidence in myself, because for the first time you are there as the person responsible, making every decision, and I made them. I didn't chicken out of them — and you can very easily do that. You can just call up your attending and say, well, what do you think I should do . . . I wasn't reluctant though I was a little scared. But I wanted to take on the responsibility because I knew that if I didn't take it on now, I'm going to chicken out of it every time; it's going to be no different. (Interview, Elite.)

Though most residents ultimately reached a point of satisfaction with their general expertise and ability to act and make independent decisions, their sense of confidence did not apply equally to all skills. Confidence in different techniques varied, and was related to the amount of experience the resident was able to accumulate in each procedure. Confidence in obstetrical ability seemed to surpass that in gynecological ability, partly because of the way in which the skills necessary to conduct a successful childbirth were defined. "Ob is pretty cut and dried. Catching babies, no big deal; whereas there is little more variability and unexpectedness in gynecology." (Interview, Elite.)

Because of the lack of training in oncology, none of the residents felt capable of performing radical surgery unaided.

> There are some things I wouldn't feel confident to do, I wouldn't take on myself. I would have someone who is more specialized or who knew the operation better. Most of the operations I think I could do with no trouble. Radical surgery I wouldn't tackle. (Interview, Elite.)

In general, residents also lacked confidence in their ability to perform surgical operations that required intervention into organs surrounding the tubes, ovaries, and uterus. This was due to the anatomical limits imposed on gynecologists. A fourth-year resident explained:

> I would have to get help for surgery for carcinoma. If I had to do an internal iliac ligation, I couldn't do that myself. If I had to dissect out ureters, I couldn't do that. If I had to repair a bowel, I couldn't do it myself. (Interview, Elite.)

In many ways Mass Hospital was the antithesis of Elite Medical Center. Unlike Elite, where residents were exposed to a combination of obstetrics and gynecology during all four years of training, at Mass the program was divided into two parts, with the first eighteen months spent exclusively in obstetrics and the second eighteen months exclusively in gynecology. This structure gave rise to a number of problems.

First, services were not hierarchical in the sense that one member was more experienced and skilled and could act as a role model, teacher, and supervisor. Instead, residents at similar levels of training were clustered together on the same services, often with no senior resident from whom to learn. The situation was exacerbated by the lack of attendings available for supervision and teaching. The problem was most acute in obstetrics, because residents were less medically experienced in general in their first year of residency, and particularly on the labor row, which served as a port of entry for new residents.

> I have never been supervised very closely. I remember the day I came here. They said, "Have you ever done a delivery?" And I said, "Yes I have done some at home," and they said, "OK, go deliver the patient and if you have any problems call me." And that was it. I didn't know the routine; what sort of sutures they use in this hospital. I used the ones I wanted to because that was what we were using back home and nobody came to teach me how to do it.
>
> [Q. You could do fifty deliveries and still be doing them incorrectly?]
>
> Right, but how do I know that the other resident is teaching me the right way anyway. He may have gone through the same thing I am going through. (Interview, Mass.)

Unlike Elite, residents at Mass did not have the option of a gradual transition to new roles and responsibilities. The abrupt nature of the role change, the feeling of technical incompetence, and the lack of supervision resulted in a general state of anxiety among junior residents. The anxiety was increased by the knowledge that when a problem occurred in obstetrics it was usually an emergency, which required quick action.

> You are just left alone; you are just left alone. And when you realize that you are in trouble, you can ask for help but you know it may take many calls. It takes many questions, like "What do you think is wrong here?" and "Why do you think that you can't wait?" And they make you make decisions that you really can't make because when you are asking for help, it is because you really need it . . . you are playing with death and besides you have two patients, you have the mother and the baby. You can lose both of them or either one of them. (Interview, Mass.)

> I worked the labor row last year and every time I got off the elevator, it was like walking into a time bomb, because you didn't know what was going to happen when you opened that door. It can be very quiet one minute and

> pending disaster the next, and the anxiety up here can get to you because even when it is quiet, you are just waiting for the catastrophe. (Interview, Mass.)

The situation was even more acute during the evening and night hours, because the small attending staff went home and the residents had to rely on "obstetrical associates"[5] for answers to questions and approval for and assistance with surgery. This suggests an interesting paradox in the training experience at Mass. Though residents were forced to assume more responsibility than they were capable of handling early in their training, they were never allowed to make a final, independent decision. Residents were critical of the fact that chief residents couldn't "even approve Pitocin stimulation, let alone a cesarean section. You can't learn to take responsibility if you are never given the chance." (Interview, Mass.) Only an attending and some obstetrical associates were allowed to approve surgery.

One obstetrical associate was supposed to sleep in the hospital each night and be on call for emergencies. However, they rarely, if ever, remained in the hospital overnight. Residents continually told me that "associates don't sleep in the hospital and often they can't be reached by phone or it takes too long to reach them and they don't come to see the patient and they give the impression that they don't want to be bothered." (Field Notes, Mass.) The fact that advice, if obtainable, was usually given by phone was also disturbing to some residents. One resident said, "Most of the time when you call an attending . . . and you ask him to make a decision . . . he doesn't see your patient. And medicine is something, if you don't see the patient, you cannot always give the right judgment." (Interview, Mass.)

The problem facing a resident confronted with an emergency after 6:00 P.M. was not only locating an attending or associate for advice, but locating someone with the authority to approve surgery, if it was indicated, who would also agree to come to the hospital and be present during the operation. Obviously, there was a time lapse, and in obstetrics this could result in a disaster.

The situation at Mass was serious for yet another reason. Because it was a public institution, it tended to get more complicated and problematic labors than other institutions. Although this was partially because poor people in general have poor health, it was also because Mass was a dumping ground for patients who were unwanted elsewhere, primarily because they lacked prenatal care. Since Mass, unlike Elite, could not refuse treatment, there was almost always a problem on the labor row. When women in the high-risk category were on the labor row, residents held their breath and hoped their shift would end before the delivery occurred. Such was the case involving a woman with a rheumatic heart condition. One resident told me, "Everyone is afraid they will be the one who will have to deliver her. I'm glad when it is time to get off and I hope she will deliver while I'm not here." (Field Notes, Mass.)

Exactly how residents were able to learn under these circumstances was a puzzle to me. One obvious possibility, of course, was that they didn't learn very much and left the residency as they had entered it, lacking skill and knowledge. However, it did not appear to be true that senior residents were incompetent. Even the residents themselves were not quite sure how they learned, but they did offer some possible explanations.

Occasionally, Mass residents were able to get someone more experienced to demonstrate a difficult technique.

> The time I had a second twin and I did my first internal inversion, I had a senior resident there. I just told him I want to do an internal inversion, you have good experience, so I want you by my side. Don't get scared, just let me do it. If I can't do it then I will tell you to do it, and I did it. But I had him by my side. (Interview, Mass.)

Especially conscientious residents used outside resources to fill in gaps in knowledge.

> We were at the same level and there wasn't much going on from one side to the other. So for my part, I did a good job. I attended most of the conferences, like two major

> conferences a year, and I kind of made up for all the things that I missed. That was the best I could do. I didn't have a senior person around to teach something about obstetrics, high-risk obstetrics, so I just selected all the conferences so that I wouldn't miss anything. (Interview, Mass.)

A more common experience seemed to be that residents learned in part through the sheer volume of patients they handled and in part through their own errors. When an outcome was unsuccessful, the resident knew to change his technique the next time a similar problem presented itself.

> Most places will have one or two of something and we will have thirty of them. Also we get to manage our cases much more by ourselves than you get to do in other places. In a lot of places residents can't do forceps without an attending . . . If you don't learn enough, you are going to mess up. I mean with all the stuff that comes in you've got to make decisions about. If you aren't on the ball and don't pick up on the stuff, you are going to have some real disasters, and they will put so much pressure on you that you will have to learn something. (Interview, Mass.)

> One day you find somebody who tells you this is this, then the next day you find something that you think is similar, until the day that you say, "I don't have any doubts." How do you know that this head will get through the cervix and this one is high and won't? Most of the time you don't need anything but your fingers and what you see, and you see a lot here. (Interview, Mass.)

> How did I learn? The same way you learn everything in this hospital, through your mistakes. And if there is something you really can't do and you know you need help, you have to get on the phone and call ten people to come here and help you. (Interview, Mass.)

Errors did occur and were often due to the residents' lack of skill and inability to obtain assistance when problems arose.

Sometimes they were errors of omission, indicating both a lack of skill and a lack of the confidence a resident needed to act quickly and independently.

> Well, there are many sections done and the patient doesn't need it. The patient probably didn't need it ten hours earlier, but when you have a labor that wasn't induced properly, then you need the section because then you have the patient there arrested with ruptured membranes for such a period of hours. You can't just wait ten or twelve more hours and at that point you know you should have done something earlier. Until that moment you didn't realize it; for the next patient you will know. Or the attending will come over and tell you, why did you wait so long and I will tell him, why weren't you here to tell me not to wait so long, I didn't know that I was waiting too long. (Interview, Mass.)

Some of the errors were discussed at great length during residents' meetings or at grand rounds. Much to the detriment of Mass patients, residents frequently learned what should have been done after the fact rather than before.

By the end of the eighteen months, residents were saturated with obstetrics. As one resident told me, "The only thing I want to do is not have to do any more time up there. You get to do everything; you have more complicated ob than you can handle." (Interview, Mass.) However, because residents had no experience with gynecology during the first eighteen months, they were totally lacking in confidence as gynecologists, though they did have confidence in their ability as obstetricians. As one resident explained, "I'm going on my third year here and I have had only two weeks of gyn." (Interview, Mass.) The result was an uneven sense of accomplishment and a professional identity heavily weighted toward obstetrics.

> Well, you see when you finish eighteen months in ob, you are supposed to feel like an ob . . . Well I felt incomplete.

> I just finished ob but I wanted to finish gyn too. (Interview, Mass.)

> Well, you feel confident in ob when you are a senior in ob, and you feel confident in gyn when you are a senior in gyn. But the way we have it here, when you are a senior in ob and feeling competent in ob, you are still feeling incompetent in gyn. (Interview, Mass.)

The amount of supervision in gynecology was slightly better than in obstetrics. The situation also produced less anxiety in residents because the nature of gynecologic problems is fundamentally different from that in obstetrics. In gynecology, a great deal, perhaps the largest part, of surgery is elective, which means that it does not require immediate attention and can be scheduled at the surgeon's and patient's convenience. Furthermore, only rarely do emergencies occur in gynecology, whereas they frequently occur in obstetrics.

Attendings did examine surgical patients preoperatively and had to approve all surgery. By rule, an attending was supposed to be present during the surgery as well. Residents, however, were frequently frustrated in their efforts to find an attending who would scrub with them. If the chief resident was available, he could scrub on one case. However, since two services were scheduled for surgery during the same time period, one service was always lacking a supervisor. Residents often spent afternoons on the phone trying to locate a willing attending, and cases sometimes had to be canceled when they failed.

Another disadvantage of the dearth of attendings was that the same few tended to scrub with residents most of the time. Unlike Elite, where residents were exposed to a variety of surgical techniques because of the variety of attendings available for teaching, at Mass residents were exposed to a relatively limited selection of techniques. Since Mass attendings were drawn largely from former Mass residents, variety was further limited. Some residents saw an advantage to this situation, as one resident explained.

> The thing I like best about Mass is that the attendings let you do it your way. If you want to do a certain surgical technique and it isn't the attending's choice, he will let you do it. It is a tradition. We have problems with attendings who were trained elsewhere because they want you to do it their way. Mass is good because it allows you to experiment with procedures and techniques. (Field Notes, Mass.)

According to residents, the rule that an attending be present in the surgical suite was often modified so that an attending needed only to be present somewhere on the surgical floor.

> Show the attendings that you are good, the moment they trust you around here, you are free. From that point on most of your contact with the attending is by phone except for good tough cases; otherwise it is more just to get an opinion . . . With surgery it is the same thing. The moment they trust you, they know you are a good surgeon, that's it, you assume the whole responsibility. When you start they are there.
>
> When you get to be an intermediate or senior, you take over the surgery. They won't scrub with you but they are in the room or the coffee room . . . In gyn it is mostly the last six months of your training when you start operating and supervising instead of the attending. He won't scrub at all if everything is OK. (Interview, Mass.)

Part of the problem with the relaxed attitude about supervision was that there weren't any clear criteria for promoting residents from junior to senior status. Often promotion depended more on departmental need for coverage on a service than the resident's ability. Periodically, in obstetrics when coverage was needed on labor row, an intern would temporarily be promoted to resident status so that he could order drugs. Likewise, in gynecology several residents were advanced from junior to senior status in surgery after only three months of experience, thus making each supervisor of his service.

> [Q. You were chief after only three months?]
> Yes, usually you aren't chief after three months, but we don't have senior people to be chief.
> [Q. Are there any criteria for being chief, like doing so many cases? Who decides?]
> It just depends on circumstances. The Head decides when you are going to be chief.
> [Q. And it has to do with need for coverage?]
> That's right.
> [Q. Is Dr. X. on your service?]
> He was earlier, but now he is on another service and he is chief there.
> [Q. And both of you had the same amount of gyn experience?]
> Right, but you can learn what you need to know in two or three months and then you have to call an attending before you can do surgery, so that makes it OK for the patient. (Interview, Mass.)

In the same way, the rule prohibiting residents from doing vaginal surgery until after they had had six months of experience with abdominal surgery was also circumvented.

> There are some rules down on the ward. They say you aren't supposed to do vaginal hysterectomies until you finish six months in gyn. But it is up to the senior resident. If I want to give it to the second year, if they have had practice before in ob-gyn, then I can give it to them. If you think the other doctor is able to do it, you can give it to him. (Interview, Mass.)

In spite of the problems, many residents believed that training at Mass was excellent for developing a sense of confidence because of the variety of pathological conditions available for them to practice on. As at Elite, confidence was related to the reduction of uncertainty through experience with a large range of such conditions.

> I think it is a very good program here to assume responsibility and especially to scrub with a guy and teach him while you are still a resident because that will give you full confidence and good practice. Besides, the material, like the number of twins you deliver and things that are rare here or relatively rare here are extremely rare outside.
>
> When you grasp it here, on the outside you may do it once every ten years. I delivered three sets of triplets. Because of the number of patients we see here in eclampsia, sick patients . . . we won't be bothered when we see such things in practice. (Interview, Mass.)

Another resident expressed his feelings about Mass this way:

> There are advantages and disadvantages. It's like being thrown into the water without being able to swim. You either sink or swim, and in a sense if you can get through a lot of the crises that occur on the labor row, then you build confidence in yourself. You have handled the crisis, you have met it and you have been successful at it, so you gain a little bit of confidence and the more times this happens to you, the more confident you get in your judgment and ability. If you are not successful, then it is the patient that suffers and then your ego goes right out the window. (Interview, Mass.)

By the end of the last year some, but not all, residents were able to feel a sense of confidence in obstetrics and gynecology. Some of the residents at Mass sounded similar to residents at Elite.

> I stopped calling the attending to ask him what to do with a problem. When I first started, I had to keep calling the attending to ask him what to do, but in time you manage everything yourself. The last six months you feel that you will be able to manage any problem that comes along. (Interview, Mass.)

Other residents, however, expressed a marked concern over their lack of experience in gynecology, as is evident in this remark made by a resident caught in the middle of the changes in the Mass program:

> I had the worst rotation of all the residents in the program. In the first year, I had six months on the labor row. Then I was sent to the clinic for four and a half months. The rest of the time, one and a half months, I spent in the emergency room. They didn't make the rule that a first year couldn't work in the emergency room until I was a second year. So then I spent three months straight of my second year in the emergency room.
>
> I spent three months in complicated obstetrics and I spent three months in pathology — that is, nine months and then two months of vacation, one for each year, so I finished my second year with no gyn at all. So this is the first time I'm getting any gyn, and now I have to go back to ob because they are changing the program and I have not had any gyn at all and they are sending me back to spend three months in ob again. That will make nine months of gyn. But one month of vacation makes it eight months and six weeks of oncology; that makes only about six months of gyn in the whole three year program.
>
> When I was an intern, the rule was no interns rotated through gyn, so I did straight ob and didn't get any gyn at all . . . The head of gyn told me when I was done, if I didn't feel that I had enough experience, I could stay another six months. (Interview, Mass.)

It is obvious that all residents did not emerge from training with equal amounts of practice and confidence. Insofar as no two individuals can have exactly the same experience, variation could be noted not only between programs but within programs as well. Residents at Elite had more training in endocrinology because it was a department emphasis, and Mass residents had more exposure to radical surgery because of that department's specialization in oncology.

There was variation in the actual amount of experience acquired within the same training program. Neither Elite nor Mass attempted to evaluate formally the resident's actual technical skill, although oral and written examinations were used to test knowledge. Nor were residents required to perform a certain number of operations in order to be graduated from residency. The requirement was that a certain period of time be spent in an accredited training program. Length of time, however, does not guarantee technical expertise.

Aggressive vs. *Conservative* — *Two Approaches to Surgery*

With the accumulation of confidence and a sense of mastery of technique, there came changes in judgment as well. Residents made a distinction between two types of approaches to treatment. An aggressive orientation involved intervention, especially surgical; a conservative approach implied somewhat greater restraint.

> Well, you have a woman, let's say with an interuterine growth retardation. When should you plan to take this woman down and let's say induce her, deliver her by section? Or when should you just wait and sit on her and let her go into spontaneous labor on her own? That's conservative; the first approach is aggressive. (Interview, Elite.)

Residents seemed to shift from an aggressive to a more conservative orientation toward surgery once they became satisfied with their technical experience.

A number of factors influence a physician's decision-making process. The nature of available professional knowledge, the unique characteristics of the patient, the individuality of the practitioner, all influence judgment.[6] During a resident's training, situational factors, in addition to increased surgical sophistication, affected his judgment. That is, his need to practice surgical techniques influenced the way in which he perceived, and assigned priorities to, all the pieces of information before he came to a decision. When what he wanted was technical experience, he tended to adopt an aggressive approach, usually some form of surgical intervention.

> A patient with an x ray that is borderline, she may be cephalopelvic disproportion, she may not be a cephalopelvic disproportion. Well, just because she has a figure of 200, which the book says is cephalopelvic disproportion, do you section her because of the x rays, or do you let her labor a little bit and see if she will deliver from below [vaginally] without causing any damage to herself or the baby? That's the difference. You are weighing your therapeutic approaches and there can be a very aggressive way to do things.
>
> Every time you see a complication or a pathological dip [on the fetal monitor] you section her. Well, nobody is really going to dispute you, but is that really doing the right thing? I've learned; before, I used to be aggressive. When you are young you want to cut, you want to do forceps, you are more aggressive. As I have become older and more experienced I have become more conservative. When you are younger you want to do the sections; you have no experience whatsoever and you want to do sections. So you see some dips and you say, "Oh, my God, she needs a section." You are colored by those approaches; that's all part of training. After you have done a lot, you don't need that technical experience, so then your judgment, your clinical judgment, comes into play and you say to yourself, "Well, maybe we should wait a little bit longer." Or sometimes by being so aggressive you hurt the patient. You have either done harm to her or to the baby. It doesn't happen often, but when it does, it really sticks in your mind and that tends to make you conservative. (Interview, Elite.)

Surgical intervention in childbirth can be motivated by other factors. From the obstetrician's point of view, surgery is a quick solution for difficulties encountered in labor.

> Some people may tend to cut quicker around her than to sit on the patient . . . It's a problem; I got to get rid of it . . . let's operate. If I section her, I don't have to worry about it. You know what I mean. (Interview, Elite.)

At Elite, the residents claimed that attendings, who were supposed to be role models, occasionally allowed personal factors to affect their judgment.

> In ob . . . you have aggressive modalities at hand, and sometimes being aggressive is easy. It may not be the best thing to do, but it is the easiest approach and the quickest and may be influenced not only by medical judgment but also by your own personal attitude at the time, which happens here. Like a party that night — a section because he is having a barbecue and he is doing the cooking. It happens; you know it happens. Or, "I don't particularly like this patient and I'm not going to sit up all night with her." Just horrible to me and my way of thinking; that's just horrible. (Interview, Elite)

> As far as doing cases goes, you have to look at it in two ways. First, is this case indicated, and second, when it is indicated, how do you go about doing it. Probably as far as indications for cases go, certain chief residents on the ward service have better indications, because sometimes I have the feeling that the private attendings are doing cases for financial reasons. When it comes to doing the case, the private attending with all the years of experience can teach you a lot more of the actual surgical techniques than a fourth-year resident can.
>
> [Q. The attendings may have financial reasons at heart when they look at indications for surgery, but wouldn't

> the chief resident, especially if he was aggressive, interpret those indications in terms of the experience he needs?]
>
> Right, but we know it [reason for surgery] when he says it; he says it outright. He is honest about it. He says, "Well we know that this case is not really indicated but we are doing it just for teaching purposes, to do it." An attending will never admit to anything like that. He always says, "This is an indicated case; this lady has to have her uterus out." So you will never learn from him when to do or not to do a hysterectomy. (Interview, Elite.)

Changes in judgment could be observed in other aspects of the resident's work. Forceps were used more frequently by first-year residents than they were by senior residents, who had mastered the technique. A first-year resident explained:

> Well, there is that gray area of prophylactic forceps in which I use them a lot to gain the experience of using them. There is almost no time when you can't use them, unless the woman delivers before you get the forceps on. (Interview, Elite.)

In contrast, a fourth-year resident said, "I rarely use forceps now. You know, when I was a new resident we used them quite a bit to get the experience. But I don't think they are necessary most of the time." (Interview, Mass.)

When the need to practice surgical skills was combined with a lack of patients presenting pathology that matched the resident's need, the tendency to stretch the limits of judgment was even more tempting.

> Sometimes in gyn, there are women who come in for hysterectomies. They are D & C, possible hysterectomies. I know I am going to get the hysterectomy, but there are some women that just don't need the surgery and I go for the D & C and say, "Well, this might hold her for the

> year; it doesn't feel like a big mass, it doesn't feel too irregular. Why don't we wait to see what happens to it?" There is no reason to do the surgery at this point in time. When you are not hungry for cases, you don't have to be dishonest about it, but a few times it has happened. (Interview, Elite.)

When residents reached the point where they were satisfied with the amount of surgery they had performed, when they had gained confidence in themselves and were reasonably sure they could handle most problems, they tended to be more conservative in judgment and to pay greater attention to patient needs. At that point, social factors were given more consideration. A fourth-year resident explained:

> I am cooler and stopped pretending that I am a big surgeon . . . You get a little more conservative in managing patients. I suppose in time we learn the social aspect also. The first thing when you start residency, you want to do more surgery, you want to be a great gyn surgeon. When you have done your surgery, you look a little more personally at your patients.
>
> Like if I did an ectopic when I was a first year, I would just go in and take the tubes, the ovaries, and everything to stop the bleeding. But now I would see her tubes and try to be a little bit more conservative and think this patient may want a baby in the future and look at her more as an individual than when I started. (Interview, Mass.)

Was the shift toward a conservative orientation permanent? Possibly the urgency of mastering surgical techniques and reducing uncertainty was so compelling that residents acted against their other values, which were restored once the pressure of training was relieved and residency completed. For some this explanation was probably true. Yet it doesn't explain the unnecessary surgery that also occurs in private practice, by surgeons no longer in need of training, in such quantities that the hysterectomy has become one of the two most frequent operations in the United States.[7] An alternative explanation suggests itself. If the Elite and Mass programs were representative of training in obstetrics and gynecology in general, residents, in addition to learning technical operative techniques, are encouraged to value surgery over prevention or well care, and also are exposed to attitudes and rationalizations that excuse occasional questionable surgery for personal gain. Some residents, not all, expressed a casual acceptance of unnecessary surgery. A fourth-year resident told me:

> I have done cesarean sections on private patients under spinal anesthesia and the attending knows that it is a so-so indicated action, but he figures if he turns the case to the resident, it is indicated. I have done several sections where he says, "You do the section" and then he looks at me and says, "Now don't you think it is indicated?" I have said nope, but I did the section.
>
> I would justify it for teaching purposes for myself and financial gain for him. Patient said yes, he talked her into it, it's OK with me. But I tell him [attending] right off, this is not indicated. (Interview, Elite.)

Perhaps, then, the attitudes the doctor acquires in residency are not shed but continue to influence his behavior in private practice. If this is so, surgical training itself is contributing to the proliferation of unnecessary surgery in obstetrics and gynecology.

Notes

1. See Chapter VI.
2. See Chapter IV.
3. Joan Stelling and Rue Bucher, "Vocabularies of Realism in Professional Socialization," *Social Science and Medicine*, 7 (1973), 664-665.
4. Renée C. Fox, "Training for Uncertainty," in *The Student Physician*, Robert K. Merton, George Reader, and Patricia L. Kendall, eds. (Cambridge: Harvard University Press, 1957).

5. Obstetrical associates at Mass were physicians who had completed residency but had relatively fewer years in private practice than the attending staff.
6. See Gary Burkett and Kathleen Knafl, "Judgment and Decision-Making in a Medical Specialty," *Sociology of Work and Professions,* 1 (1974).
7. See Chapter IV.

VI

Negotiating to Do Surgery

I HAVE ARGUED that residents emerged from training with different amounts of practice in surgical skills. The amount of experience or practice a resident had in what he defined as important skills was significant in determining not only his actual level of ability, but also his confidence as a surgeon. Simply stated, residents sought the opportunity to gain experience. This chapter will illustrate how this was accomplished within the social context of training and the effect these efforts had on patient care.

Formal policies of hospitals and the medical profession set limits on the kinds of acts in which physicians can engage. In spite of formal rules, most forms of organization tolerate variation within a range of quasi-legitimate behaviors. This is true also of medical training. Residents developed a group perspective in which questionable acts were justified because they were interpreted in terms of their usefulness as learning experiences. To some extent, residents had to negotiate for the opportunity to carry out these acts.

Residents believed that those among them who went through training complying with formal rules gained less experience than residents who intervened on their own behalf and who could negotiate and bargain for access to certain types of work and patients. At Elite and Mass, residents used the term "aggressive" to mean "the ability to intervene successfully on one's own behalf." Aggressive residents, it was believed, were more successful in gaining experience.

> An aggressive resident is one who places himself in a position so that he is able to accomplish and observe and do those things he wants to do, as opposed to a more quiet guy who doesn't make his presence known and who sort of gets lost in the shuffle . . . I think that perhaps I'm more aggressive than some. I know how to get more out of relationships than some do. I'm a finagler; I mean I can always make it a point to come out smelling good . . . I think I can control my environment a little more than some can. (Interview, Elite.)

The object was to control others' actions so that personal goals could be accomplished. To some degree, a resident's ability to control was related to his year of training; senior residents had important advantages that junior residents lacked. However, at every level of training, residents were engaged in a process of negotiation and bargaining that involved attendings, colleagues, and patients. At Elite and Mass, though residents' acts and behavior differed because of differences in the training institutions and programs, the twofold objective was the same. Residents negotiated for a position in which they could optimize the opportunity to do work that was defined by them, at any point, as contributing to their professional development. At the same time, they attempted to decrease or avoid work that they did not perceive as making a similar contribution. It will become apparent that the needs of patients were often secondary to the residents' own needs and that cooperation on the part of the attending staff was often necessary in order for residents to accomplish their goals.

Getting Cases Turned

Securing the opportunity to do some types of work required negotiations between residents as well as between residents and attending staff. This was so because attendings had an important power over residents: they had the authority to permit or deny residents the opportunity to perform surgery. Therefore, doing surgery was often related to the resident's ability to gain the cooperation of an attending physician.

At Elite, residents had two types of surgical-training experiences. Ward gynecology was taken in the second and fourth years and involved performing surgery on institutional patients under the supervision of a fourth-year chief resident. Private gynecology was taken in the first, second, and third years and involved performing surgery on private patients under the supervision of an experienced surgeon. Basic operative skills and techniques were supposed to be learned in private gynecology and perfected in ward gynecology.

Learning surgery in private gynecology was predicated on the assumption that attendings, under most circumstances, would turn their surgical cases to the residents to perform — that is, would allow residents to do the surgery. Residents believed that unless an individual was hopelessly incompetent or the case was too difficult for the individual's level of skill, the most senior resident on the operating team should be allowed to do the surgery. Residents frequently complained to me that it was unjust of attendings to refuse to give them their surgery. Attendings, they believed, were obligated to teach residents and not just use them for scut work. Residents were willing to do scut work because they expected to be rewarded with cases. When the reward was denied and cases were withheld, it was considered a serious breach of faith.

Attendings had reputations based on their willingness to turn cases, and most of them turned a good proportion of their surgery. Those who did not turn cases were universally disliked and, if possible, avoided by residents. This, of course, means that surgeons in hospitals that train residents frequently do not operate on their own patients, although they do sign the operating room record, are legally responsible for the outcome, and receive the surgeon's fee. One resident remarked, "When a surgeon says he has done a thousand operations of a certain type, it means he has scrubbed a thousand times." In the beginning of my observation period, several residents voiced concern over my knowledge of this practice. They believed the public wasn't aware that surgeon substitutions routinely operate in teaching hospitals. Apparently they were correct, because when the television program "60 Minutes" ran a story on "ghost surgeons," the public reacted with alarm.

• • •

For most major obstetrical and abdominal gynecological surgery, the basic surgical team consists of three actors. The principal actor is the surgeon, who is attended by first and second assistants. On the patient's right stands the person occupying the surgeon's role. The first assistant stands across from the surgeon on the patient's left. The surgeon makes the decisions, but the first assistant is also actively involved with the surgery. The second assistant stands to the left of the first assistant and is not actively involved in the surgery, usually doing little more than holding the incision open with an instrument called a retractor.* Assistant positions are sometimes filled by specially trained surgical technicians, but in teaching hospitals residents perform these functions as part of their training.

The three positions on the surgical team were not equally valued by residents. The most valued was that of surgeon; the person occupying that role was most active and assumed more responsibility than any other member of the team. The role of the second assistant was most disliked; as residents described it, the main function was to "hold a retractor" and "watch surgery from a bad angle." Furthermore, because the second assistant doesn't play an active role in the surgery, a resident occupying that position didn't have an opportunity to demonstrate his ability to the attending. A first-year resident explained the significance of this:

> If you are anything less than a first assistant on a case, the doctor will never really know how much you know. But if you are a first assistant and by the grace of God things

* The team's placement is reversed if the surgeon is left-handed.

> seem to go all right postoperatively and you take interest in watching his cases . . . [the attending physician] begins to see that you exist. And if you show some technical expertise — and that is all surgery is; it really has nothing to do with anything else — then he is more apt to let you do something. (Interview, Elite.)

Surgery is learned through apprenticeship. At Elite this meant that for major surgery, second-assistant positions were usually occupied by first-year residents; first-assistant and surgeon positions were more likely to be occupied by second- and third-year residents. The goal of all first-year residents was to maneuver a first-assistant position; second- and third-year residents attempted to secure for themselves the position of surgeon. This situation generated a considerable amount of negotiation among residents as each jockied for a position on the surgical team.

When a case was turned, the attending scrubbed but took the position of first assistant on the surgical team. The general practice was for the attending to depart after the major portion of the surgery was completed, leaving the residents to stitch subcutaneous tissue and close the incision. The resident was responsible for dictating the official operating room record, which was later signed by the attending.

Regardless of who actually performed the surgery, the attending was officially listed on the record as the surgeon and was legally responsible for the patient. Because of malpractice problems, the surgeon, of necessity, had to take into consideration the expertise of the resident whom he allowed to do his surgery.

Residents, however, believed that attendings used personal criteria to decide whether or not to turn a case. At Elite, where there was considerable opportunity for informal interaction between residents and attendings, residents thought that personality was as important as skill when it came to their getting cases.

> Well you look pretty, you're able to talk to the attending in a nice way. It is a very personal thing. I have seen it

> with all the residents here. The only guy I saw that got a lot of cases they didn't like was Dr. X. because he was an exceptionally good surgeon. So they would give him cases even if they didn't like him. (Interview, Elite.)

The chief administrative resident explained it this way:

> It has to do with personality and how hard you work from the beginning and your attitude when you first start the program. You put out for doctors down in the labor room. It starts then, way before you ever get into the operating room. When you are chief, it takes working up the patient [taking medical history, ordering tests, and so on], doing the surgery, and then following up the patient every day of the week. I made rounds on every Saturday, Sunday and holiday, and there was a note on every chart of every patient that I operated on . . . and you have to do good surgery and there is an et cetera element of schmaltz, bullshit. It's the game whether you are in ob-gyn or medicine or any other profession. You can be a lawyer and still need the schmaltz and do the little things — it's anywhere to get ahead and get your training. (Interview, Elite.)

New residents felt they had to prove themselves to attendings before they would be allowed to do anything "meaningful" in surgery. Residents who rotated through the private gynecology service in the latter part of their first year had a greater chance of getting cases because they had been exposed to the attendings during their time in obstetrics and thus had had the opportunity to make a favorable impression. A first-year resident explained:

> I was unfortunate because surgery was my first rotation and no one knew me and I had to prove myself. This is a common problem in medical education. It is supposed to be advanced education and the burden of proof is always on the individual. Before he is given responsibility or before anyone makes an effort, you know, to go out

> and do something for him . . . Unless you have the skill, they [attendings] aren't going to let you actually do the case. But to develop the skills, tie knots and retract, I think there is a lot of personality involved in letting you get started getting involved. (Interview, Elite.)

It is probably accurate to say that both factors, informal relationships and skill, were important criteria. How much skill a resident needed, however, was relative.

Lack of skill alone did not prevent a resident from getting a case in surgery. In fact, a case was not always turned to the person most capable of doing it. For example, when one of the second-year residents who had had surgical experience before coming to Elite scrubbed with the third-year chief, the attendings always turned the case to the chief, who, though he had less skill than the second-year resident, was not judged to be less skilled than would be expected of one at his level of training. A person's position, not his expertise, was important. Residents were expected to be inexpert at what they were doing. In general, once a resident had mastered a skill, he stopped practicing it. He would try to progress to something more complex and pass the unwanted task to someone who needed the experience.

However, when the resident's lack of skill was greater than what might reasonably be expected for his level of training, he could be punished by being allowed to do less of the attending's surgery. The fewer the cases a resident was given, the less skillful he became in relation to others at his level of training. This in turn further reduced his future chances of getting surgery from attendings. The result was that his original lack of skill became the barrier to acquisition of the skill he needed.

This is a serious flaw in surgical training. Although the vast majority of surgeons are well trained, it is also true that the incompetents, even though they may be small in number, are rarely removed from a training program or from the profession. In training programs, especially where there are private patients who might sue their surgeons, residents may be allowed to continue but will be given minimum opportunity to perform and thus master difficult tasks. Such surgeons are graduated and certified and are free to practice surgery without constraint. The public, in turn, not only does not know who these surgeons are, but does not have access to the technical knowledge with which to assess medical and surgical performance.

Manipulating Surgical Assignments

At Elite, though the attending maintained ultimate control over the surgical situation through his right to deny cases, the third-year chief resident occupied the status on the team that carried with it the expectation and the informal right to do the attending's surgery. However, the type of experience a chief had during his third year was related to the type of experience he had had during the previous two years. If he had encountered difficulty getting cases before, he would experience difficulty getting cases in his third year.*

In spite of this potential difficulty, the third-year chief did possess an advantage junior residents on the service did not have. The third-year chief made the room assignments in surgery, which meant that he decided which surgeons the residents on his service would assist. Thus, the chief resident constructed the surgical team and could decide the type of cases on which he himself would scrub as well as the surgeon with whom he would scrub. In making the assignments, he was aware of several conventions that would be followed. If a case was to be turned, it would go to the most senior resident on the team, regardless of his actual technical ability. Since the

* The situation was considered so serious that one resident, beginning his third year after the changes in the program requiring two third-year rotations in private gynecology, petitioned to be relieved of the second private gynecology rotation. He contended that since he had not been allowed to do cases in the past, he could not now expect to get them, and he refused to spend six months of his third year "holding a retractor." His petition was successful.

resident to whom a case was turned did not usually have the option of turning it to a more junior member of the team, when a chief decided to scrub on a case the surgery was performed either by him or by the attending.

In the position of chief, the resident assessed his own operative needs and then chose the case and the surgeon that would best meet those needs. Thus, each chief resident had different criteria for choosing the surgery on which he would scrub.

One chief, who had encountered difficulty getting cases in his first two years of residency, was more interested in observing technique than in actually doing the case. He explained:

> I don't just want to scrub with anyone. I just want to scrub with a few people that I am really going to learn from . . . If I know a guy has a good technique and there is something he can offer me when he is doing a case, I would rather go with him because I won't see such a thing all the time. Catch it from him and do it another time. (Interview, Elite.)

A more typical strategy was to scrub only with those attendings who the chief resident knew would turn the case and only on those cases he believed he would benefit from doing.

> You just come out and ask him, "Are you going to turn that case to me," and if he says no, you scrub with somebody else. You know the attending men want senior residents to scrub with them because it is easier for them to have a good assistant or to assist someone who is good, and if they aren't going to turn the case and there is another case that you think you might be able to do, then you tell them that you won't scrub with them. There are certain attendings that you don't want to scrub with anyway. You let somebody else scrub with them [your junior]. You pick the cases you want to scrub on. (Interview, Elite.)

The expectation was that the chief would place himself, for most of the time, with an attending who would allow him to do the surgery. It was not expected, nor did it often happen, that the chief felt a responsibility to see that his juniors on the service got a share of the surgery. Rather, it was believed that a junior's opportunity would come in his third year, when it would be his responsibility to make full use of a chief's advantage. A fourth-year resident explained:

> They [juniors] will have the chance to get whatever cases they want next year. You know it's gradation; if you aren't going to get the case, then they aren't going to get the case. Or if they aren't going to get the case anyway, then you might as well scrub and get the case. If you are pretty sure whoever it is isn't going to turn them [the junior residents] the case, then you might as well take it yourself. I think that is the way most of us feel because there are plenty of cases to do by the time you are done. (Interview, Elite.)

Depending on the attending and type of case the chief chose for himself, a number of possible outcomes emerged for a junior resident. From the junior's point of view, the most desirable chief was one who had accumulated a considerable amount of practice in his junior years and now needed to master the more difficult surgical techniques and therefore would choose for himself only complicated abdominal surgery and vaginal hysterectomies. (These types of cases were usually reserved for the third and fourth years; consequently, junior residents didn't expect to be given the opportunity to do them.) Under optimal conditions, the junior resident who was working with a chief who chose only complicated cases could expect to do surgery a good bit of the time. Whenever the junior resident was told to scrub on a simple case, such as a technically uncomplicated hysterectomy, without the chief and with an attending who had a reputation for turning cases, he could reasonably expect to be allowed to do the surgery, as long as his technical skill was up to expectations for his level of training. The problem was that some chiefs, especially those who lacked experience, were more likely to scrub for any case, simple or complicated, they believed they had a chance of doing. When this happened, a junior resident was forced to scrub either on cases too difficult for him to do or with surgeons who had reputations for not turning cases. Under these circumstances, a junior resident would get to do very little surgery.

As a result of these variables, junior residents experienced greatly different kinds of training during the year. One resident reported a very good experience in which he had the opportunity to do a satisfactory amount of surgery.

> You have to understand you are dealing with private patients. The attendings are being paid for treating these patients. You can't ask an attending to give a case when he doesn't trust the resident. He is tense, he doesn't want coronary spasms all the time because he feels this resident is not confident enough to do the procedure. Then he [the resident] is going to struggle a lot and may make a lot of mistakes, like clamping a ureter or something else that can really harm the patient. [In the first year] you scrub with them [the attendings] in sections and deliveries and they know what you can do. I mean they know if you are aware of the things that need taking care of.
>
> Another thing is, even if you don't get the case, you follow up on the patient. Then the attending knows that this is a guy they can trust. So once they get this confidence in you — that you know the technical part and you take care of the patients and they think they can talk to you socially — then they give you the case. I know, for example, if he [an attending] is in a hurry, he isn't going to give me the case. That never bothered me because I got fifteen hysterectomies in private gyn in the second year, which is very good. (Interview, Elite.)

In contrast, another resident got to do only one hysterectomy in private gynecology during the entire year.

> In private gyn, I didn't do very much because they [the attendings] didn't like me. In the second year, you can't choose the cases you want to scrub on. You are left with whatever is left, so you don't even get a chance to scrub on many. Then it depends on how much they like you whether you are going to get to do much. I didn't even scrub on ten hysterectomies in ten weeks in the whole private gyn. I did all the peritoneoscopies. I didn't even scrub on the major cases. (Interview, Elite.)

During their first year, residents reported universal dissatisfaction with the private gynecology rotation because they had to do most of the scut work. Since only two major cases were scheduled at one time, a first-year resident was almost always forced to second assist regardless of where he was sent to scrub. If the first-year resident was sent to scrub on a minor case that neither the second- nor the third-year resident wished to do, he might be allowed to first assist, depending on the attending's evaluation of him. However, as long as the second- or third-year resident wanted experience on minor cases, the first-year resident would be unable to perform an active role in surgery. An angry first-year resident rotating through private gynecology after the program was changed explained his problem:

> The two third-year residents on the service didn't get much experience during their second year because attendings wouldn't turn them cases. Now they are scrubbing on cases that they know they won't get instead of only scrubbing on cases that they think they will get. This prevents the first-year resident from getting to first assist on cases which are not going to be turned because the third-year resident first assists. Regardless of which room the first-year resident goes to, he ends up second assisting. (Field Notes, Elite.)

First-year residents had virtually no control over their situation and no power over more senior residents and attendings. Not only were they unable to choose the cases on which they would scrub, but they had no one beneath them to whom scut work could be delegated. As one first-year resident put it:

> When you get to the point where they can turn you cases, then you should also be at the point where you scrub with the person you like so that you by-pass all the people you don't like and you give them to somebody on a lower level. I mean, that's what happens. You give the first-year person all the dregs and you take the best cases. (Interview, Elite.)

On the private gynecology service, especially for junior residents, relationships with other residents as well as rapport with the attending staff were important in determining how actively one would be allowed to participate in surgery. The resident's schedule determined who his chief would be, and the explicit hierarchical nature of the service meant that the chief exercised considerable power over those under him on a particular service. Those who learned to manipulate the scheduling system during their first year and intervened when schedules were made out for the second year reported greater satisfaction with the year in general. One resident explained:

> I didn't say anything; I just took my schedule as it came. Some people did manipulate that and I think because of that they got to do more than other people did. I was the last one to find out you could manipulate. I didn't know you could do it. I just thought it came automatically out of heaven. Then I found out and I was unhappy with some of my rotations. (Interview, Elite.)

The same hierarchical structure existed on Elite's ward surgical service; the chief had a great deal of influence over the training of those under him. There was, however, one major difference having to do with the type of patient serviced. Unlike private patients, institutional patients were regarded as teaching material. The expertise of the resident performing the surgery, therefore, was not so critically evaluated as when a private patient was involved. In the matter of ward cases, the most significant factor from the junior residents' perspective was who the chief was.

The principal function of the ward surgery service for the chief was to provide whatever surgical experience he had not been able to obtain on the private surgery service. If a resident had been prevented from doing surgery during his third year and, as a result, was still somewhat inexperienced, he would attempt to maximize his exposure to surgery in the fourth year, when he became chief of ward gynecology. In this capacity he had control over the ward service and the right to do any case he could find, but without the benefit of close supervision from a more experienced surgeon. As a consequence, less skilled residents did more surgery on institutional patients without the benefit of tutelage and supervision. The more skilled residents received a larger proportion of their training on private patients under the guidance of an experienced surgeon. When I mentioned this to one of the residents, he responded, "That is what the ward service is for. You gain experience on institutional patients." (Field Notes, Elite.) For the institutional patients this meant that more surgery was being performed on them by less skilled and sometimes unsupervised residents.

In addition to allocating cases, the chief had another important function. The chief of the service worked in the clinics and selected the surgical cases. An "aggressive" chief would "find" more cases from among patients in the clinic than a chief who was not aggressive. A chief who was still interested in doing surgery himself or who felt some obligation to meet his juniors' need for experience would also be more likely to find cases than a chief who had temporarily lost interest in surgery.

The case-juggling at Mass was similar to ward gynecology at Elite, although junior residents had an advantage over their counterparts at Elite because they didn't have to rely on their chief to find cases. Juniors could locate their own cases because they worked in the clinic as part of their gynecology rotation. The problem at Mass was slightly different. The chief was supposed to be present in surgery to supervise the juniors on his service. However, if the chief had lost interest in surgery, he would attempt to reduce the amount of surgery performed on his service. One senior resident, who was especially uninterested in doing surgery, frequently gave away his operating room time to other services and gave away cases to friends on other services. This behavior aroused considerable anger in the juniors on his service, who felt they were being deprived of needed surgical experience.

Obtaining Approval for Surgery

Another important source of control that attending physicians at both institutions had over residents was their authority to grant or deny permission to perform surgical procedures on institutional patients. Because the hospitals were legally responsible for the residents' acts, department rules at Elite and Mass mandated that an attending's approval be obtained for all obstetrical and gynecological surgery, except the most routine, and for all drug-induced or -stimulated labor. Residents at both institutions worked under the same restriction, and the negotiation and bargaining for surgical approval was similar.

At Mass, in spite of the lack of supervision, the rule regarding surgical approval was strictly enforced. At Elite, however, residents seemed better able to stretch the rule. If the resident was willing to accept total responsibility for his act, the surgical-approval rule could be circumvented. Because of the increased responsibility, senior residents and chiefs of services were more likely than were junior residents to proceed on a case without approval. When the rule was circumvented and the outcome of the case was satisfactory, the resident was safe from censure. However, if the rule was circumvented and the case went badly, the resident was in jeopardy. Since circumventing the rules placed residents in a vulnerable position, several factors entered into the decision-making process.

The type of case under consideration was a factor. In general, if the problem was considered routine, such as stimulating a labor, or the indications were clear, such as the need for a repeat cesarean section, the resident would often proceed independently and inform the attending at some later, more convenient time. Under these circumstances, even the rule that an attending be present in surgery might be circumvented. A third-year chief in obstetrics explained his procedure:

> What I have been doing is telling them after the fact. I say, "Oh, Dr. So-and-So, I have been pitting [giving the patient Pitocin] the patient for the last couple of hours. I wrote down that you agreed with what I said . . ." In theory there is supposed to be an attending present [in surgery] but practically it's "Oh, by the way, we had a ruptured ectopic [ruptured Fallopian tube due to a tubal pregnancy]. Do you agree with what we did?" So there is a lot of autonomy. (Interview, Elite.)

When the procedure was major or the surgical indications were ambiguous or questionable, residents, especially if they lacked confidence, were more likely to protect themselves by following the rules. Another obstetrical chief explained:

> Before I did a cesarean hysterectomy, which is a major procedure in which you are essentially sterilizing the woman, that was always cleared. Postpartum hysterectomies were always cleared. But if I wanted to do a section for a prolapsed cord or a section for an abruptio, I would make all the arrangements, make the decision myself, then I would call my attending and say, "Look, I have such and such a case, I want to do this, what do you think I should do," knowing all the time what I wanted to do. Very big things or sometimes esoteric things, where I wasn't sure, every time that I felt I wasn't very confident, I would go for a consultation. (Interview, Elite.)

As the above statement suggests, residents at both Elite and Mass made a distinction between asking an attending what to do with a case and telling him what had been done or was planned for a case. In spite of the fact that an attending was being consulted, as long as the resident knew what he wanted to do, he saw himself as making an autonomous decision. A Mass resident explained:

> I don't know; it's kind of funny around here. You can get an attending and do just about anything, really. I mean, most residents go to an attending that way. The resident knows what he is going to do; he has made up his mind. He is just getting verification from the attending. (Interview, Mass.)

In the same way that attendings evaluated residents in terms of their skill and judgment, the residents evaluated attendings. Attendings were not seen as being equally competent, so their advice was not equally valued. An Elite resident commented:

> I suppose over four years you get to know what different people have to offer; some have a great deal to offer positively. Others have very little to offer. You find out which surgeons are skillful with their hands, like Dr. A., who you try to emulate surgically; who thinks well on his feet, like Dr. B. (Interview, Elite.)

Mass residents also evaluated the attendings.

> There are a few attendings that when they say something to me, I get another opinion because I figure, oh, oh. Now someone else could tell me something and it would sound just as bizarre and I would do it because I have confidence in them and I figure if they tell me wrong, they can still get me out of it. Through experience I have seen what their judgment usually has been and I judge whether they know their subject. (Interview, Mass.)

Attendings were sought for different reasons, depending on the resident's needs and his evaluation of the attending's ability. An Elite resident explained: "In my own mind there are some people that you listen to because you respect their judgment, and then there are some people that you have to go to just because they are on the service." (Interview, Elite.)

If a resident felt he needed assistance with a difficult case, he would try to choose an attending whom he respected. However, if the resident simply wanted approval for a procedure he had already decided to do, he would try to choose the attending most likely to give him the approval. Because surgical indications are not based on absolute criteria, attendings sometimes had different opinions regarding the amount of pathology necessary for surgery to be approved.

> You are talking about cases that we take that are borderline, and borderline, you can go up or down . . . A fibroid, which is the most common operation, if it is twelve-week size, it will depend on how the attending feels — if it is big enough or not, if you do a twelve-week fibroid or don't do it. (Interview, Mass.)

After working with attendings for a period of time, residents knew what individual attendings were likely to approve. When they had a case, they attempted to seek approval from the attending most likely to cooperate.

> Like for cystic hyperplasia, Dr. A. sometimes won't [give approval] but others will. But then it depends on the patient, too. And sometimes for a vaginal hysterectomy, Dr. B. is hard to get an OK from but Dr. A. will. (Interview, Mass.)

If, in spite of all precautions, an attending did not cooperate, residents frequently "shopped around" until they found an attending who would agree with them. At both Elite and Mass, shopping was a common strategy for getting to do what you wanted to do.

> If the resident is fairly sure about what he wants to do, he calls the attending and tells him and the attending says

> yes or no. If he is wrong or you don't think he is right, then you ask somebody else . . . On clinic cases you are in charge and if the attending doesn't agree, then you just go to another attending who will agree with what you want, if you feel that strongly about it. (Interview, Elite.)

At Mass, in obstetrics, surgery was sometimes approved over the phone by an attending who didn't come in and examine the patient. If the attending happened to be unfamiliar with the resident who was making the request, he would instruct him to have an associate examine the patient before granting approval. One of the residents on the labor row remarked, "Basically, they [attendings] aren't listening to what you are saying, just who is telling them. In the past your judgment has been OK and on that basis they figure your judgment is OK this time and they just OK it." (Interview, Mass.)

Since the person approving the surgery usually didn't see or examine the patient, a resident could, if he desired, describe the case in a way that would increase the probability of his getting approval.

> You shop around to get somebody that is going to agree with you. I mean we all do that, make a diagnosis and, in effect, if an attending is not here, unless you are way off base, he has to go along with you because, after all, you have seen the patient and you are right there. He is only getting what you are telling him over the phone, and by telling him only certain stuff, you can sort of do whatever you want to do, which is bad and good, I guess you know. (Interview, Mass.)

At Mass, in the gynecology division, an attending did see each preoperative patient. On Monday morning, residents from each service presented their surgical patients, who had entered the hospital the night before, to an attending. The attending, in turn, would examine the patients and then, without the benefit of the results of preoperative tests, would approve or deny the surgery. Some weeks several attendings appeared for this ritual, but at other times only one attending was present. With only one attending in attendance, shopping was not possible. Since residents could not ignore the approval rule, they developed another strategy to handle the situation.

> The resident brings a patient in and if the attending says no to surgery, they send her home and bring her back into the hospital in a few weeks and get a different attending to see the patient and they will probably get an approval. (Field Notes, Mass.)

This practice illustrates several important points. Residents would have been unable to manipulate to the extent they did if surgeons were in greater agreement about what constitutes sufficient symptomatology and pathology to warrant surgical intervention. Moreover, the inconvenience to patients, who often had to make elaborate child care arrangements, only to be sent back home and then called in again a week later, was of little concern to many residents, who cared only that surgery was available for them.

Residents who, in addition to mastering the art of manipulation, were also able to develop a good relationship with a few attendings were best equipped to maneuver teaching experiences to their own advantage. For example, residents sometimes needed the assistance of a cooperative attending physician to secure certain rare types of surgery — surgery that was frequently referred to as teaching cases. One such operation was the cesarean hysterectomy.

According to residents, there are two methods for treating a pregnant woman who needs a hysterectomy. One is to perform a cesarean section and a hysterectomy at the same time. The indications for this surgery are quite rare, because not only must the pathology be adequate to warrant a hysterectomy but the candidate should also have had a previous cesarean section. If she has not had a previous cesarean section, a vaginal delivery is possible, followed somewhat later by a hysterectomy. This operation, a postpartum hysterectomy, is generally regarded as better for the patient because "most people think that the morbidity and trauma are much more with a cesarean hysterectomy than it is in a postpartum hysterectomy." (Interview, Elite.)

In spite of its rarity, most residents were able to do a couple of cesarean hysterectomies.

> This year as chief [of obstetrics] I would like to do as many cesarean hysterectomies as possible. I don't want to do cesarean sections; I want to do cesarean hysterectomies. I don't want it [private practice] to be the first time, and I need this — I don't say hundreds of cases but a few cases — to build up my confidence. (Interview, Elite.)

Although the risk of morbidity and mortality increased for the patient, indications for cesarean hysterectomy were sometimes stretched and the surgery approved. "Well, if a patient has a carcinoma in situ or fibroids or you can talk them into it for sterilization, you can extend your indications; you can redefine indications." (Interview, Elite.)

In order for the resident to do the case, an attending had to approve the surgery. If the indications had been stretched, the justification was for teaching purposes.

> Well, if your attending on service happens to be on your side and says, "OK, for teaching purposes we will do it," then all you have to do is talk a woman into saying she doesn't need her uterus after she has her baby. Why not do a cesarean hysterectomy on you. But then she probably should have had a previous section. (Interview, Elite.)

A similar procedure might be performed on a woman who wanted an abortion and either has pathology sufficient to warrant a hysterectomy or has been persuaded to have a hysterectomy as a method of permanent sterilization. An Elite resident who did seven of these procedures explained it this way:

> I did a lot of hysterectomies when I was chief of obstetrics because my attending was nice, aggressive, friendly, and he wanted me to be exposed to almost everything possible. So when I was chief of obstetrics, I did seven hysterectomies postpartum and on pregnant ladies that had fibroids and wished abortions and also wished permanent sterilization, which made it a perfect setting for a hysterectomy . . . Otherwise they would have to have a suction curettage to terminate their pregnancy and a tubal ligation or a hysterectomy six weeks later . . . A lot of people say no because it is a slightly bloodier procedure. That's the only disadvantage in pregnancy . . . I still think that a pregnant uterus is very easy to operate on because at that time all your fascia [fibrous tissue] and things are just beautiful. You just go zip along. (Interview, Elite.)

Finding "Material"

The single most important resource in training, from the resident's view, is the patient who presents a medical problem that corresponds to the resident's need for experience in a particular skill and who agrees to undergo surgery. The residents at Elite and Mass believed that a prerequisite of successful training was the ability to locate patients and to convince them that surgery was in their best interest.

At Elite, residents looked for patients primarily in the various clinics administered and staffed by the department. The chief of ward gynecology was expected to spend two afternoons a week in the clinic "looking for material." Some residents went to the extent of arranging their third-year schedules so that their clinic rotation preceded their labor room rotation. This was done so that they could look for potential cases from among the women who would deliver while they were in obstetrics. They were hoping most of all to find candidates for cesarean hysterectomies. One resident explained:

> You have to look for the kind of person in the clinic and if you don't have that rotation beforehand, you have to

> hope that the person in the clinic is looking for you, because once she gets into the hospital — once she is in labor — it's difficult to talk someone into a hysterectomy. (Interview, Elite.)

Another source of surgical material was the evening family planning clinic. Aggressive residents tried to work as many evenings as possible to enlarge their range of patients seen and increase their probability of locating pathology.

At Mass, the clinic was one of two major sources of cases. Because all three services occupied the same clinic space and all of the residents on each service were looking for their own cases, competition often reached an extreme. For example, if the clinic coordinator happened to assign one service more than its share of postoperative cases, residents complained: someone who just had surgery wasn't a potential surgical case. There was so much competition that some residents felt the clinic was worthless as a source of cases. By the time a patient reached the clinic, she either had a clearly nonsurgical problem or she was postoperative.

> You go to the clinics and everybody tries to get the operating cases, so by the time they reach the gyn clinic, they are usually postoperative. Sometimes they are first visit. They have a reference from another doctor and they come to the clinic. You examine the patient, they need surgery, OK. But most of the time you don't get much from the gyn clinic, so you have to go to other clinics like family planning, like the emergency room. In the family planning clinic, they come for birth control and they have five or six babies and maybe a prolapsed uterus or incontinence, so you take the case. (Interview, Mass.)

Many residents believed that the emergency room was the most fruitful source of cases. At Mass, the emergency room functioned as the main examining and intake area of the hospital, and patients were seen there before referral to a clinic. As a result, a resident who worked in the emergency room had first choice over all the patients who used the hospital. Residents could increase their case load by working in the emergency room during the night shift and on weekends when the regularly scheduled resident was off.

Every resident had to spend three months in the emergency room as part of his second-year rotation. Following this rotation, residents usually returned to one of the gynecology services. The resident faced the dilemma of knowing that when, in two or three months, he would be on the gynecology service, he would be very much in need of cases, but here were the cases passing through his hands while he was in the emergency room. The solution was what the residents called "saving cases," instead of referring them to the resident on call or to the clinics, as the rules stipulated.

> I worked in the emergency room a month ago. I was assigned there but I wasn't in the hospital at the time, so if I sent the patients to the clinic, I would miss them. So you keep the names and telephone numbers and say I will call you. Of course, if it is an emergency, you have to admit the patient. If it is a fibroid uterus, it can wait for a couple of weeks. (Interview, Mass.)

Some residents were unaware of this practice and naïvely sought the most expedient solution for the patient. One second-year resident explained:

> If you have a rotation in gyn before you go to the emergency room, you learn the tricks. If you just go to the emergency room, you just want the patients to be taken care of, and you think when your time comes, you will get your cases and you just look for the betterment of the patient because you don't know that the patient can wait for a week or two without any problem . . . You can just as easily save the patient for yourself. Say a patient comes in with a fibroid uterus; the patient doesn't need surgery right away, the patient can wait. Most people keep their names and give them a call and tell them to come to the

> clinic when they know they will be there. But these things you only know after you have had a rotation in gyn. (Interview, Mass.)

Often, because gynecological surgery is elective, and waiting would not imperil the woman's health, residents told patients that the hospital was full and they would be called as soon as there was space. In this way, residents could accumulate a large number of cases. One resident proudly showed me twelve pages of names he had collected in six weeks in the emergency room.

Selling the Hysterectomy

After a potential patient was located, she had to be persuaded to have surgery. As one resident put it:

> You have to look for your surgical procedures; you have to go after patients. Because no one is crazy enough to come and say, hey, here I am, I want you to operate on me. You have to sometimes convince the patient that she is really sick, if she is, of course, [laugh] and that she is better off with a surgical procedure. (Interview, Elite.)

One important skill residents acquired during their four years' training was that of talking women into agreeing to surgery. Since surgical indications were sometimes questionable, persuasion became an important skill for a resident to have. When there was no indications at all, surgery was not approved. However, when minor pathology was present, indications were sometimes stretched and surgery approved. An attending at Mass announced at a residents' meeting, "Doing cases in residency that aren't indicated because you want to do a few cases while you are still in training is not OK when the indications are way off." (Field Notes, Mass.) In other words, surgery was permissible as long as the indications weren't "way off."

Besides the practice of performing hysterectomy for sterilization,* another abused form of gynecological surgery was hysterectomy for small, benign, asymptomatic fibroids, which can disappear without surgical intervention or remain intact without symptom. I asked residents what they would do with nine-to-ten-week-size asymptomatic fibroids and received the following answer from a fourth-year resident:

> Uh, most likely I would do the surgery. I will offer the woman, you would probably offer the woman, you would explain the situation. I don't think it would be right to say you have a horrible disease or you have cancer or anything like that, I have to do this surgery.
>
> I would explain to her that she has fibroids that are nine-to-ten-week size, that she isn't going to have a family anymore, she doesn't want a family anymore, that these fibroids *may* some time in the future grow bigger, *may* get symptoms, *may* cause her trouble, she *may* need surgery at some point in time, and if she would like to have surgery done now, it can be easy surgery, vaginally. As a consequence she won't have any more children, but she won't have any fibroids and she won't have any potential for disease.
>
> [Q. Put like that many people would say yes.]
>
> Right, but is that being dishonest?
>
> [Q. Those fibroids may also disappear by themselves.]
>
> Right, but you are only saying they may do this or they may do that and essentially you let the patient make up her mind. Usually when patients hear they have fibroids and there is some bleeding, there is a sufficient symptomatology. (Interview, Elite.)

A resident at Mass explained it this way: "Well, you stretch a little bit a minor indication but no major indication. For exam-

* See Chapter IV.

ple, a sterilization in those patients over thirty-five with mild pelvic relaxation, you could stretch the indications for a vaginal hysterectomy." (Interview, Mass.)

After spending months in the clinics and emergency room listening to residents talk to women about surgery, I saw a pattern emerge. The residents' tactics, based on high volume, were similar to that of any effective salesperson, regardless of the product; that is, the greater the number of contacts, the greater the probability of making a sale. This type of high-turnover sale was especially suited to the high-volume, quick-turnover conditions in the clinics and emergency room. Like any sophisticated salesperson, a resident could judge within minutes whether a woman was going to buy a hysterectomy. When it appeared that she wasn't, he used another tactic. Many women came to the clinic simply to obtain birth control and were completely unaware that anything was going to be found amiss. Residents believed that women would eventually accept surgery if they were given some time to think it over. Thus, after a resident had completed his pitch and the woman was still reluctant, he would tell her that he would call her in a week and discuss the surgery further. The woman was dismissed and the next prospective case was brought into the examining room. The entire interaction, including physical examination, usually took three to four minutes.

The sales pitch used by residents at both hospitals was remarkably similar; in some cases the very same words were used. The resident opened by moving from a general problem for which a number of solutions, including doing nothing, were possible, to the solution he was going to try to sell, usually a hysterectomy. The more supporting evidence that could be brought to bear on the problem, the more secure the resident was in his pitch. The pitch frequently began when a woman over the age of thirty-five requested birth control or permanent sterilization in the form of a tubal ligation. If, in addition, the resident could locate evidence of some pathology, he would attempt to sell a hysterectomy. Essentially, the resident was substituting a hysterectomy (surgery he wanted to do) for a tubal ligation (surgical scut work). The tactic was similar to the "bait and switch" technique used in sales in which the advertised item is discredited and another, more expensive, product is substituted in its place. For example:

> Dr. W. saw a woman with a class III Pap smear. He explained to her that it could be a precancerous condition, in which case surgery was indicated, or an infection, in which case medical treatment was indicated. Then she told him she had eleven children and wanted a tubal ligation but had fibroids so that it couldn't be done. In that case Dr. W. told her it was even more likely that she should have a hysterectomy. (Field Notes, Mass.)

> Dr. S. examined the woman and then told her that her uterus had slipped a little and it would be best to take it out. He told her that eventually she would have problems with it. It would press on her bowels and she would be constipated. She was told that it should come out through her vagina and they wouldn't have to cut her stomach. (Field Notes, Mass.)

> Dr. Z. told her she had moderate dysplasia and if she thought about having her tubes tied, then she should think about a hysterectomy because that was the only thing that would really cure her. (Field Notes, Mass.)

My observations indicated that clinic women were never advised of the relative dangers or rates of complication of the vaginal hysterectomy versus the tubal ligation. Instead, residents stressed that the vaginal hysterectomy was easier than the abdominal hysterectomy because "you don't have to be cut." Even if this statement were true, the reasoning is dishonest, because the real comparison is between the vaginal hysterectomy and the tubal ligation.

When the pathology involved a fibroid, "the tumor" was presented in such a way that the woman would initially become alarmed. Later, when the resident assured her that fibroids weren't cancerous, the psychological impact had already been made. Many women were frightened into surgery by the word "tumor," which is closely associated with cancer and death in our health-conscious society.

> Dr. Z. told her she had a tumor in her stomach and that while it wasn't an emergency, she should have it out as soon as possible. He said, "It is not cancer but there is a possibility of small cancer tumors within it." (Field Notes, Mass.)

After fear and doubt had been planted in a woman's mind, the next step was to discuss the purpose and utility of a uterus. These discussions illustrated the residents' basic disregard for the female reproductive tract, which they saw as functional only for childbearing.

> He told the woman that the only function of a womb was to carry a baby, and with a tumor [fibroid] she couldn't get pregnant so she might as well have it out. (Field Notes, Mass.)

> He told the woman that a uterus was only needed for babies and that her problem could turn into cancer in five or ten years, and to guard against it, she should have it out now. (Field Notes, Mass.)

> Dr. P. told the woman she didn't need her womb, that it was only a cradle for the baby, and if she wasn't going to have children, she didn't need the cradle. (Field Notes, Mass.)

The next step in the pitch was to assure the woman that a hysterectomy would not reduce her femininity, attractiveness, or sex drive.

> Dr. S. told the woman that ovaries make you feminine, the vagina would stay, and sex drive would be the same. She just wouldn't have a uterus. (Field Notes, Mass.)

> Dr. W. told her that a hysterectomy wouldn't make her any less a woman, that she would still have a sex drive,

> but she wouldn't have to worry about things anymore. (Field Notes, Mass.)

Finally, the pitch was concluded with a summary of the "advantages" of a hysterectomy and the promise of a simple, quick operation.

> Dr. S. explained to her the advantages of a vaginal hysterectomy: no more periods, no fear of cancer, no loss of sex drive, the operation would only take twenty-five minutes, and she would probably have to have it out sooner or later because of the fibroids. (Field Notes, Mass.)

Once the woman agreed to surgery, she lost whatever power she previously had had — the power of refusal. The situation changed from one of negotiation to complete control by the resident. The patient was expected to trust the knowledge and wisdom of her doctor. She was not consulted on the form her surgery would take nor was it expected that she was capable of understanding medical-surgical mysteries. The resident, influenced by his own need for practice, decided what operation he would do. Women were not aware that there was a choice.

> You might have a borderline, say ten-to-twelve-week-size uterus, and rather than doing it from above [abdominally] you can do it from below [vaginally] and do a little bit more difficult vaginal hysterectomy but hopefully not increase the morbidity for the patient. You have an older woman who has a pessary in with a fourth-degree prolapse, you may want to do a LeFort [sewing the vagina closed] on her. Namely, because it will be good for her condition and otherwise because you have never done a LeFort before. You know, you have that option. [Laugh.] You disagree with me? (Interview, Elite.)

Likewise, women were not consulted on the type of childbirth experience they would have. Residents exercised the option to use forceps until they felt confident of their technique with them.

Once the woman was in the operating room and her abdomen was open, residents tended to want to remove more than just the organ originally bargained for. A healthy appendix or ovaries were sometimes removed.

> Occasionally we do an appendectomy, but occasionally you could be in trouble doing an appendectomy at the same time you are doing other surgery. To do an appendectomy when the appendix is well, usually, most of the time it doesn't increase morbidity. It's a preventive measure. (Interview, Elite.)

"Prophylatic" appendectomies became so frequent at Mass that the department ruled they could not be performed without the approval of the head of the gynecology division. Appendectomies performed while tubal ligations were being done were especially censured.

Not all residents used all of these techniques to the same extent. The extent to which they were used, however, was, as we have seen, closely related to the amount of surgery the resident wanted to do and only marginally related to ethical issues. Most of the residents condoned these practices if the surgery was done for training purposes, and, for the most part, many attendings complied. From Chapter V, we know that once a resident became satisfied with the amount of surgery he had performed, the patient's interest received more consideration. However, until the resident developed a sense of confidence in his ability to perform a particular surgical technique, his need for practice was a salient influence on patient care.

Avoiding Work

In order for the residents to achieve what they regarded as a successful training experience, it was necessary for them not only to secure desirable work but to avoid scut work, work involving skills already mastered. Attending physicians who by reputation did not usually turn cases and patients who possessed characteristics or pathology that residents found not to their liking were also to be avoided.

At Elite and Mass, the most common avoidance technique was dumping, described in Chapter V. When a resident had a relatively higher status than others, he would dump undesirable work or uncooperative attendings on a more junior resident. Senior residents, because they more often held positions of high status, were better able to dispose of work and attendings than were junior residents.

Another method of avoiding unwanted work was to discourage women from undergoing certain procedures — or at least to refrain from encouraging them. These procedures always involved routine skills the resident believed he had mastered.

> Dr. X. mentioned to me that there was a gravida 14, para 13 in the labor room and she didn't want a tubal ligation. He said many of the women are afraid tubal ligations will affect their sexual functioning and it needs to be explained to them. However, he said, from a resident's point of view, a tubal ligation is a nuisance because there is nothing new to learn from them after you have done a few. So if the woman says no, they don't push it because they don't want to do them anyway. (Field Notes, Elite.)

At Elite, some work was avoided to such an extent that an important medical service was not available to patients. This was the case with abortions. Although numerous first- and second-trimester abortions were performed by attendings on private clients, they were not available to the residents' institutional patients. When questioned about the lack of an abortion service for institutional patients, the hospital staff reported that, for religious and moral reasons, residents could not be required to perform them. On questioning residents, though, I found that with few exceptions all of them planned to offer abortion as a service to their patients in private practice. Either residents didn't have convictions preventing them from performing abortions, or the desire for financial reward was greater than their convictions. It should be noted that first-trimester abortion involves dilation and curettage, which is one of the skills acquired very early because it is used to treat a number of uterine conditions, abortion being one. When I probed further, residents finally told me, "We don't learn anything from abortions. All you do is insert a drug and wait. Residents want to do things they learn from." (Interview, Elite.) Another resident said, "Well you see, this is the whole point. We are residents; we don't get anything out of abortions; we don't learn anything from it. It's a pain in the neck." (Interview, Elite.)

It was also to the resident's advantage to avoid some individual patients. At Elite, "undesirable" patients could be transferred elsewhere, usually Mass, where residents did not have a similar option because the institution was legally bound to treat all who came to its door. Thus, Mass was known at Elite — and elsewhere in the area, I'm sure — as a dumping ground for unwanted patients.

At Elite, residents frequently referred to some women as "Mass patients." The term was used to denote women who presented a trait or a combination of traits residents disliked, including certain pathology, physical features such as obesity, attitudes, and kinds of behavior.

At Elite, patients in the terminal stages of cancer were frequently transferred to another hospital, usually Mass, where, they were told, there were experts to handle their problems. This was accurate, but it was also usually true that part of the motivation was to dispose of dying patients who were going to require a great deal of care. One night, for example, an elderly woman with terminal cancer was brought to the emergency room by her family. The resident on call asked the family to return the next day, when the chief of ward gynecology could examine the patient. The resident on call explained that if he admitted a patient like that to the ward gynecology service without the chief's approval, the chief would hate him every day until the woman died. The next day the woman was transferred to Mass. (Field Notes, Elite.)

Patients who came to the emergency room requiring what

was viewed as scut work were also transferred to Mass if possible. One resident explained:

> A considerable number of ladies come in with incomplete abortion or vaginal bleeding. Now if we accepted all those cases, we would do nothing but D & Cs all day and night. A certain percentage of those patients need to be transferred. (Interview, Elite.)

At Elite, where residents had to do most of their own scut work, avoiding patients who required such work was attempted whenever possible. To the residents, a labor room filled with women who were not in active labor but nonetheless required care was such a situation. A woman who came to Elite in the early stage of labor but had not received prenatal care there was told to go to Mass for her delivery. The Elite resident would then contact a Mass resident and explain that their obstetric beds were full, which, of course, Mass residents were unable to check. When the woman was one of Elite's own, she was made an offer she couldn't refuse: she would be told that she could remain in the hospital, in bed with a needle in her arm, prevented from eating, drinking, or smoking, or she could go home and return when her labor was active. Women usually went home.

Mass residents didn't have the option of transferring patients. Patients, however, could frequently be avoided through stalling. Often this was done when the resident was unsure about treatment and couldn't arrange for a consultation with someone more experienced. Residents on the labor row told me they could evaluate the ability of the resident on the shift before their own by the work that was left undone or decisions unmade when they arrived.

Another method of stalling involved postponing treatment until the resident knew he would be off the particular service. A patient could be given a Band-Aid-type of remedy and asked to return to the clinic at some later date. This method was used in the infertility clinic at Mass.

> Infertility clinic, there aren't any attendings. There is supposed to be but he doesn't come very often. Most of the residents don't like endocrinology because you have to read — they like surgery. So the residents have a two-month rotation in the endocrinology clinic and the patients have been coming for five or six years. They keep coming and the resident knows that in two months he is going to be off the rotation. So the resident tells them to take their temperature and wait for lab results and he gives them an appointment to come back in two months when he is out of the clinic. (Interview, Mass.)

Referral to other clinics within the hospital was another stall tactic. At Elite patients on whom nobody wanted to operate might go through several stalls before finding a chief who would handle their case.

All of these tactics facilitated the residents' personal objective: performing the type of medical task, usually surgical, that would contribute to their skill as surgeons. In a very real sense, residents' training was incomplete until these tactics had been mastered. It is reasonable to suggest, as I did earlier, that the attitudes learned while in training continue to influence the behavior of surgeons in private practice. It is not surprising that surgeons perform unnecessary operations. After all, they are trained to do it.

Equally serious is the lack of concern and the disrespect residents learned to display in dealing with patients. Human beings are entitled to considerate treatment and good health care, but "material" is a commodity that can be manipulated and exploited for personal gain. Even if residents did change when they reached private practice, the women I observed and the poor who must receive health care in institutions like Elite and Mass would continue to be victims.

VII

Strategies for Change

By the opening decades of the twentieth century, male obstetricians and gynecologists had secured a monopoly in the health care of women. Having eliminated lay competitors such as midwives, the new experts could claim exclusive medical access and control over the organs of female reproduction. Vested with the authority of the medical profession, and unrestricted by outside regulation or competing providers, the specialists were free to create their own definitions of female health. Often these definitions have included the assumption that women are improved by castration and prophylactic hysterectomy.

Consistent with the surgical orientation established by nineteenth-century male midwifery and pelvic surgery, modern resident training in ob-gyn emphasizes surgery rather than primary care, a policy that promotes the financial and professional interests of physicians. However, when surgeons, rather than generalists, are produced in numbers sufficient to meet women's health needs, which are vastly nonsurgical, the result is a situation favorable to high rates of surgery. The belief that female reproductive organs are expendable equipment, dangerous and dysfunctional outside of childbearing, continues to provide justification for aggressive surgical practices. Thus, both attitudes and the situation in obstetrics and gynecology are conducive to unnecessary surgery.

Unnecessary Surgery: Individual or Professional Deviance?

Why is there unnecessary surgery in obstetrics and gynecology? Individual misconduct is one possible explanation. By performing unnecessary operations, certain surgeons violate professional norms. In contrast to their colleagues, these physicians are "deviant." Because they do violate the norms of their profession, nondeviant physicians might be expected to monitor and control their rule-breaking behavior.

An alternative explanation views unnecessary surgery as a manifestation of professional misconduct. Rather than violating the rules, the action is consistent with the norms of the profession. Thus, from the perspective of an outsider, the profession as a whole is deviant. In this situation, physicians would not be expected to regulate their colleagues' behavior, since it is inconsistent with the norms of the profession to do so.

Recently two sociologists, M. David Ermann and Richard Lundman, formulated a theory of "organizational deviance"[1] to explain institutional misconduct: corporations and government, like individuals, are sometimes deviant. According to Ermann and Lundman, a deviant action that is organizational, not individual, must be supported by the norms of the organization while simultaneously violating the expectations of outsiders. Such violations are most serious when they disrupt the flow of benefits to those who have a legitimate claim on the organization.

Service "organizations" like the medical profession must satisfy the question: Who should benefit from the existence of the organization? Although the primary beneficiaries of professional efforts in obstetrics and gynecology are presumed to be women, the historical and contemporary emphasis within the profession indicates a consistent pattern of goals intended to promote the interests of physicians over patients. This contradicts the publicly held medical goal of delivering superior health care to women. Organizational deviance exists when internal goals contradict publicly stated goals.

Organizational actions are also deviant when they betray client trust and violate client expectations. The betrayal of client trust is particularly evident in obstetrics and gynecology, where the pursuit of goals that promote professional interests results in policies neglectful of women's total health care needs. An aggressive surgical attitude toward the female reproductive organs is a betrayal of women's trust, as well as a violation of patients' expectations regarding appropriate physician behavior.

The most crucial distinction between individual and organizational deviance rests on whether the action, considered deviant by outsiders, is also a violation of the internal operating norms of the organization. When organization members as well as the administrative elite support a deviant action or behavior, organizational deviance exists. Since this type of deviance is particular to the group, participation by newcomers is not automatic. It results from socialization, a process in which individuals learn the rules of behavior of the group.

We have seen that surgery like prophylactic hysterectomy is accepted by physicians. Arguments supporting similar practices appear in best-selling medical textbooks and in professional journals. To the extent that Elite Medical Center and Mass Hospital are typical of training institutions, surgical training presently fosters rather than discourages unnecessary surgery.

At both Elite and Mass, residents were encouraged to acquire a medical identity linked to the surgeon's role. They vied for the opportunity to do hysterectomies and learned to respond to childbirth as if it were a surgical problem requiring intervention with drugs, machinery, and tools. Like other surgeons, these residents enjoyed operating, and their professional satisfaction was derived mainly from the surgical activity. Moreover, though surgery and superspecialty medicine were practiced with enthusiasm, well and preventive care were perceived as the least satisfying and challenging aspect of obstetrics and gynecology.

At both Elite and Mass, surgical training included a process in which residents learned the language and techniques to justify and negotiate surgery. At both institutions, consistent with the priorities of the medical profession, residents saw their first responsibility to be the acquisition of surgical skills and judgment. Patients were defined as training material and valued to the extent that their problems coincided with the residents' need for experience in a particular skill. To perform the desired amount of surgery, residents found it necessary to intervene on their own behalf, to be aggressive, and to negotiate with staff, peers, and patients. Developing techniques for talking women into agreeing to surgery was important.

Group norms regulated the limit to which acts were acceptable when done for training purposes and the manner in which the opportunity to practice skills could be negotiated. Significantly, residents condoned the idea of "teaching cases." Consequently, unnecessary application of forceps and surgery for minor pathology and occasionally on normal organs was acceptable and justified as necessary for training purposes. The attending staff offered little resistance and demonstrated their support by tacit and sometimes direct approval. Moreover, since attending physicians engaged in similar acts themselves, the example presented to residents was supportive of unnecessary surgery for personal gain. Because everyone was involved in the behavior to some extent, as long as norms relating to unnecessary surgery were not exceeded, no individual had to consider himself deviant. Indeed, the behavior was not deviant within the context of the institutions' residency procedures.

Health Care and the Poor

Unnecessary surgery and the medical maltreatment of women are symptoms of profound social problems. This book has described the disparity between the type and quality of medical services available to the middle- and upper-income classes and those that the poor are forced to accept. Because medical services tend to be delivered in the same way other goods and services are delivered, economic systems have an impact on health care distribution. In the United States a person's economic status directly affects her or his ability to secure a product or service, be it a car or a doctor. Lower income people frequently receive medical services at reduced cost and in return serve as the material for experiments and teaching. Thus, the dual health care system functions to maintain a patient population adequate to meet the needs of medical training and research.

Teaching institutions like Elite and Mass claim two goals that are viewed as complementary: service to the poor and medical training. But inside these institutions, one finds more evidence of contradictory goals as the "complementary" arrangement is more compatible with the needs of medicine than with the needs of patients.

The organization of patient services at Mass was somewhat more consistent with the special needs of its clientele than at Elite, where institutional patients were expected to utilize services in the same way as they were used by private patients. For example, at Mass the emergency room was fully staffed twenty-four hours a day and serviced nonemergency as well as emergency conditions, a necessary service for people who do not have a private physician to consult. At Elite, however, patients who came to the emergency room with nonemergency problems were received with anger by residents who were unconcerned that these patients were unable to go elsewhere for medical consultation.

Typically, institutional care is delivered in an atmosphere that is indifferent at best and often characterized by hostility, even callousness. The problem is greater than a lack of communication. Patient services designed to maximize residents' exposure to pathology spawns indifference by reducing the opportunity for a relationship to develop between physician and patient.

Statistics indicate that the poor have more illness and disability as well as higher mortality rates than the middle class. Explanations have tended to blame the poor for not using available services and resources and have also suggested that they are apathetic about their health. In *The End of Medicine,*[2] Rick Carlson argues that "caring" increases the motivation of both medical workers and patients. Thus, caring on the part of physicians is not a luxury; it is basic to good health care and may be a determinative factor in the healing process. It is reasonable to suggest that if some institutional patients appear to be apathetic about their health, the reason may be the lack of caring they are subjected to, due largely to the way in which training institutions dispense medical care.

Residents' awareness of patient rights was greater at Mass than at Elite. Nonetheless, neither set of residents regarded service to patients as the most important part of their work in residency. Patients were important only as they presented medical problems that corresponded to the residents' need for practice in a particular skill. This in turn affected the type of treatment patients received. Women in labor had to undergo numerous pelvic examinations, and their babies were frequently delivered by forceps when intervention in the natural process was unnecessary. Cesarean hysterectomies were sometimes performed when procedures with less risk of complication would have sufficed. Institutional patients were talked into having hysterectomies when the simpler tubal ligation was indicated. Once the patient was in surgery, appendixes were sometimes removed for "teaching purposes." Even the style of the operation could be dictated by a resident's need for experience. All these were done in the name of training.

Private patients are also subjected to unnecessary operative procedures. There is, however, one very significant difference. As we have seen, in training emphasis is on how incompetent, not how competent, the resident is. Incompetence is not considered bad unless it is the result of a resident's inadequate motivation. Rather, incompetence is a gauge of a resident's need for practice. Because the resident has been hired to learn, his obligation is to continue practicing a skill until he masters it. When this has been accomplished to the resident's satisfaction, such work is passed on to a resident still in need of practice. Institutional patients, as a result, are frequently in the position of receiving their care from a physician who is less than fully skilled in what he is doing. In addition to this, supervision is often inadequate, not only in the clinics and on the wards, but also in labor, delivery, and operating rooms. Mass Hospital was a case in point. At Elite Medical Center the more skilled residents learned basic surgical techniques on the private gynecology service under the close scrutiny and tutelage of an attending physician; the less skilled residents, who were refused access to private patients, learned on the clinic service, where considerably less supervision was given. Paying patients seeking a surgeon would not request the least qualified person. Yet this is often what institutional patients are forced to accept.

Elite and Mass make it painfully clear that for the poor, the cure can be worse than the disease. Not only are residents indifferent, patient services designed with institutional needs foremost, and the quality of care compromised by resident inexperience and a lack of supervision, but poor patients are expected to be grateful for what they receive.

It is obvious that physicians must be trained and that research is necessary if medical science is to advance. It is also obvious that, given a chance, most of us would avoid being the object of a fledgling physician's first experience with surgery. Yet can we justify the continued exploitation of one class of people to serve a function from which the entire population accrues such direct benefit?

The question may already be settled. With the ratio of privately insured patients increasing, some teaching hospitals are experiencing difficulty obtaining a medically indigent patient population sufficient to meet the demands of teaching and research. California physician Victor Richards, writing in the *American Journal of Surgery,* argues that surgical training will have to move into community hospitals with a private patient population.

> We are on the verge of a revolution in surgical education, for the indigent patient is vanishing from the scene and surgical education will have to be conducted in the future on the so-called "private," or "full-paying," or "insured" patient . . . The [current] system is antiquated, immoral, and socially irresponsible, yet no one will deny that it has educated outstanding surgeons, and regrettably it is hard to see how the same technical excellence can be achieved by the developing surgeon as the indigent patient vanishes.[3]

Predictably, as the involvement of "paying" patients in surgical education appears inevitable, concern about the lack of supervision in the present system will grow. Thus, despite the idea that surgical training is best accomplished by allowing residents to assume responsibility for patients, Richards argues:

> Constant unyielding prospective and immediate critical review of the resident's performance is mandatory, instead of the retrospective review which takes place after the act has been accomplished, the complication has arisen, or the patient has suffered because of the immoral abdication of total responsibility to a resident merely because the patient is unable to pay for optimal care. Education within this framework [on paying patients] requires the most tedious and painstaking supervision by the teacher, continuously and actively during the performance of service to the patient by the resident.[4]

The magnitude of violations against the poor are underscored by the concern voiced for the welfare of "paying" patients lest they be used for training purposes in the current system of surgical education.

Controls on Physician Behavior

Ermann and Lundman note that most organizations are forced to interact with other "controller" organizations that have the power to monitor and regulate their actions. The medical profession, however, has no formal controller organization composed of *lay* members. This has important consequences for consumers of medical services.

As the lay public, we have been persuaded to believe that professionalism and medical ethics always guide physician behavior. This has been used effectively to obscure consumers' need for external controls on the medical profession. As a result, regulation remains internal, in the hands of physicians. But evidence seems to suggest that physicians do not effectively regulate each other's behavior. Moreover, if behavior that consumers question is actually consistent with the norms of the profession, there is little reason to expect internal regulation in medicine, since from a physician's viewpoint, the behavior isn't rule-breaking.

When a controller organization, such as a federal monitoring agency, discovers that a business is producing a faulty product, it has the power to intervene on behalf of the public, curtail production, and, under certain circumstances, impose fines or demand consumer compensation. Government regulation may not always be very effective, but at least there are systematic and collective remedies for business practices damaging to the public good. Though health care may well be considered the most vital or consequential human service, medical consumers are virtually on their own. And patients are in a difficult position to recognize medical malpractice, since information crucial to making such determinations is largely unavailable to the public.

Essentially, the only recourse available to medical consumers against deviant practices is malpractice lawsuits. A number of factors, however, make individual legal action an inadequate remedy.

First, legal action is expensive. It is beyond the financial means of many middle-class consumers and almost totally out of reach of the poor, who are the group most vulnerable to exploitation. Second, legal action can take place only after a deviant act has been discovered. It has no effect on prevention or on detection. Lawsuits do not prevent repetitions of the behavior or ensure that future acts will be discovered. Third, and most significant, legal action against an individual has little direct impact on the profession as a whole. Malpractice suits are effective only in securing compensation for individual cases of misconduct.[5] They do not affect the quality or type of medical training, nor do they force a change of values in the profession. There is little reason to expect legal action to curb unnecessary surgery, so other methods must be considered.

Strategies for Reducing Unnecessary Surgery

Movement toward some form of national health insurance or a national health service is finally under way in the United States. With this in mind, I list several suggestions that make use of such plans as means of curbing unnecessary surgery, at least in obstetrics and gynecology.

1. Since research indicates that surgery decreases as surveillance of physicians increases, a health care plan that provides for a method of monitoring and regulating physician behavior that is more effective than the current system of professional self-regulation should reduce unnecessary surgery.

The social control of physician behavior is a complex issue well beyond the scope of this book. A model based on the system used by the government to regulate corporate practices may not be desirable in a situation where the product is human service. There is urgent need to explore new models, which include consumer involvement, for accomplishing this important reform in health care.

2. A national health plan placing physicians on a salary or based on the health maintenance organization (HMO) concept should reduce unnecessary surgery.

When health care is paid for on a fee-for-service basis, physicians make a profit from surgery as well as from illness and treatment in general. In prepaid health plans, like an HMO, where consumers are guaranteed all of their health services for a predetermined yearly fee, more money can be made if illness is prevented; surgery rates are lower because it is more profitable for the physicians not to perform unnecessary operations. However, in an HMO, because more profit can be made by nontreatment, there is the danger that important types of patient care and services may be withheld. More research on the quality of care in health maintenance organizations and prepaid health plans is urgently needed.

3. A change in the providers of medical services to women, based on a policy of greater involvement of women patients in their own health care and broader utilization of nonphysician women health workers in primary care, would decrease unnecessary surgery. It would also create the potential for a new set of health care priorities based on women's total, rather than just their surgical, needs.

The recent return of the midwife, today a highly trained and specialized nurse with several years of study and practice beyond a nursing degree, is a promising development. Nurse-midwives or nurse-practitioners can provide a large proportion of the care now delivered by obstetrician-gynecologists. It is inefficient for highly skilled physicians and surgeons who are experts in the pathology of the female reproductive organs and in high-risk pregnancy and childbirth to provide routine care, especially when trained nurse-midwives, as research indicates, are capable of handling most deliveries, as well as prenatal, family planning, and well gynecological care. Not only are nurse-midwives able to provide technical care; they bring to their work a sensitivity and concern for their clients that is lacking in many obstetrician-gynecologists.

If nurse-midwives provided most primary care, fewer obstetrician-gynecologists would need to be trained, and those who were trained would be assured of a greater opportunity to do the work they enjoy and to handle the type of medical problems for which they are trained. Since fewer surgeons would compete for the existing pathology, less unnecessary surgery should result in private practice as well as in the residency training.

The pervasive power of organized medicine is evident in many states where restrictions limit the hospital privileges of nurse-midwives, prevent them from functioning independently from physicians, and, in many cases, block reimbursement by insurance companies for their services. If nurse-midwives or nurse-practitioners are to be optimally effective, they must have a certain amount of autonomy. The traditionally strict professional hierarchy in hospitals and other medical settings has been maintained, in part, because a nurse's work supplements or assists in the central task of diagnosis and treatment, controlled by physicians. Since nurse-midwives and nurse-practitioners are trained to recognize pathology and to treat routine problems, these nurses no longer need be subservient to physicians. Nurse-midwives or nurse-practitioners can be viewed as an alternative to physicians in normal pregnancy and childbirth and in primary care. Working separately and autonomously, nurse-midwives or nurse-practitioners and obstetrician-gynecologists would provide checks and balances for each other and would offer women patients a choice in health care providers.

Health Care: A Right or Privilege?

Despite America's claim to be the standard bearer of human rights, health care reform in the United States has lagged behind such reform in many other Western industrialized countries. Perhaps one obstacle has been postponement of the inevitable decision as to whether all members of our society are entitled to the same quality of health care.

The question of whether health care should be considered a right or a privilege in the United States is far from settled. Predictably, there is strong opposition to the elimination of pluralism; it comes from powerful interest groups that profit from the free enterprise structure of medicine.

The possibility of eliminating profit in medicine and of imposing controls on the medical profession is threatening to many physicians who find the status quo in their best interest. Writing in the *New England Journal of Medicine,* Dr. Robert Sade argues against the idea of medical care as a right. Undoubtedly, there are other physicians who would agree with his position.

> The concept of medical care as the patient's right is immoral because it denies the most fundamental of all rights, that of a man to his own life and the freedom of action to support it. Medical care is neither a right nor a privilege: it is a service that is provided by doctors and others to people who wish to purchase it. It is the provision of this service that a doctor depends upon for his livelihood, and is his means of supporting his own life. If the right to health care belongs to the patient, he starts out owning the services of a doctor without the necessity of either earning them or receiving them as a gift from the only man who has the right to give them: the doctor himself . . . American medicine is now at the point in the story where the state has proclaimed the nonexistent "right" to medical care as a fact of public policy, and has begun to pass the laws to enforce it. The doctor finds himself less and less his own master and more and more controlled by forces outside of his own judgment.[6]

The decision regarding our right to health care is not one over which the medical profession has exclusive domain. As an interest group, the medical profession is just one segment of the public, albeit a powerful one. The decision will be made through elected representatives in Congress, who are charged with the responsibility of responding to the mandate of consumers, as well as the medical profession and other interest groups. Strong consumer support for legislation to establish a national health service would make it clear to legislators that Americans believe health care is a right.

A National Health Service

Although the plans currently before Congress for national health insurance would relieve some of the financial burden of catastrophic illness for the middle class, they would leave unchanged the two-class national system of health care we now have. One bill, however, drafted by Ronald Dellums (D-Cal.)[7] with the assistance of some of the original members of the Medical Committee for Human Rights, does serve as a model for equality and consumer involvement in health care. The Dellums Bill creates a national health service and attempts to guarantee basic health rights. In Dellums' view, consumers have the right to receive health care without charge or discrimination; to be treated with respect and dignity; to choose their own health providers and facilities; to have access to their own health records; to have information translated into their native tongue; to receive a full explanation on all health care questions; to have counseling and assistance on health matters; and to have access to a complaint system and to legal assistance in enforcing their rights as consumers.

The United States Health Service, envisioned by the Dellums Bill, would function as an independent agency of the federal government and be financed by a progressive form of taxation on individuals through income and on employers through payroll taxes. The service would provide comprehensive medical, dental, and mental health services without charge or discrimination to all individuals, regardless of citizenship, while they are within the territory of the United States. In addition to the treatment of illness, the Dellums Bill emphasizes health maintenance and attention to occupational health and safety. Special provision is made for health care rights of children and women. For example, the bill specifies that a woman has the right, as long as medical risk to herself and the infant does not increase the usual risk of pregnancy and birth, to deliver at home, to have at her side during labor and delivery whomever she chooses, to care for the infant at her bedside, and to feed the infant by whatever method she deems best.

In Dellums' plan, all workers, including physicians, connected with the United States Health Service would be salaried employees of the government. The structure of the United States Health Service would be four-tiered. The community, where primary care, outpatient treatment, and emergency service would be provided, is the base of the system. A community health board, elected by the community, would be responsible for all health services, including the planning of services and hiring of health workers. Districts, consisting of several communities, would contain a general hospital administered by a board selected by the community representatives. Medical centers would be located in regions comprising several districts, and services would be coordinated by regional boards appointed by district representatives. Medical centers would provide highly specialized medical services; each would also contain a health team school where all health workers, physicians included, would be trained. (Admission policies would emphasize previous health-work experience and encourage recruitment of students from the local population.) A national board, appointed by regional representatives and approved by the President of the United States, would be responsible for overall health planning. Two thirds of every board at each level would be consumers; the remaining one-third would be providers.

To protect patient rights, the Dellums Bill would establish grievance procedures and a system of health advocacy. Health advocates, with some legal training, would be employed by each community, district, and regional health board to work in health care facilities, where they would oversee patient rights and report infractions to the appropriate boards.

Legal services would be available to consumers and health workers without charge for problems related to health rights and services. Consumer and worker grievance procedures would be set up at the regional and national level.

From this brief and sketchy outline, it should be apparent that Dellums' plan would significantly change health care delivery in a number of ways.

First, it would eliminate the two-class system of health care by guaranteeing the same type and quality of services to all. In contrast to the current system, in which the grade of physician and type of facility are determined by the consumer's ability to pay, the Dellums' plan bases the choice of physician and facility on the health problem. For several reasons, the Dellums' plan would eventually phase out private medical practice as it is now known. The delivery of private health care would not be permitted in government facilities nor by physicians employed by the Health Service. Furthermore, since all Americans would automatically belong to the United States Health Service, few would opt to pay, in addition to the taxes that would fund it, the fees necessary to use private physicians and facilities.

Second, Dellums' plan would reduce much of the profit that is currently made from illness. Since there would be no need for private insurance companies, and facilities like hospitals would be run by the service on a nonprofit basis, the profit from these two sources would be eliminated from the cost of health care. The profit motive for either performing unnecessary procedures or withholding necessary ones would be reduced because physicians and other health workers would be salaried. Moreover, the expense associated with unnecessary surgery and other superfluous medical and surgical procedures would be eliminated from health care costs.

The Dellums Bill would also accomplish a major change in the consumer's role in his or her own health care. Not only does it provide for systematic enforcement of patients' rights, but consumer representatives, accountable to the community, would be responsible for health care planning. Since operating funds would be allocated to communities, districts, and regions on a per capita basis, low-income, underserved areas would have the resources to overcome their current serious deficits in health services. And to compensate for the present uneven distribution of health workers, all graduates of health team schools would be required to spend a period of up to two years working in underserved areas.

Several measures in the Dellums Bill are intended to remedy the lack of regulation and monitoring of physicians. Unlike the present medical-licensing system, health workers, including physicians, would be subject to continual competency review and asssessment. Although Dellums states the review would include supervision by users and providers of services, review procedures are not spelled out. Community, district, and regional boards, through control of services and patient advocacy, would provide some regulation and monitoring of physician conduct.

Dellums' plan, a radical departure from the current system, incorporates many of the positive features of health care systems in other countries. Some critics will dwell on cost and argue that the United States cannot afford comprehensive health care for all citizens. But the issue is one of priorities. The nation's health should be at least as important as the arms race or the exploration of space, programs for which billions have been spent. The plan is thought-provoking and controversial, and it provides for the organizational changes necessary to remove discrimination in health care. Equally important, it places regulations on health workers, including physicians, and switches the control of health care delivery from the medical profession to consumers.

A point of particular concern to the consumer is the possibility that the government may adopt a health care system in which everyone receives the type of impersonal, uncaring care now reserved for the poor. A one-to-one patient-provider relationship is a positive feature of private health care and one that is worth striving to preserve. Some clinics and prepaid plans, in which numerous providers care for many patients, reduce not only continuity of care but the opportunity for the type of bond to develop between patient and practitioner that increases humane care. Residents at Elite and Mass can hardly be blamed for their detached attitude toward institutional patients; they rarely had the opportunity to know their patients well enough as people to feel otherwise.

Changes in the structure of health care will have little impact without changed attitudes on the part of providers. In her essay "Humanization and Dehumanization of Health Care,"[8] Jan Howard lists elements essential to humane care. First, all human beings must be viewed as equally valuable. Second, each human being must be viewed as unique and irreplaceable. Third, patients must be viewed as holistic selves, not as narrowly defined medical problems. Fourth, patients' freedom of choice and full access to information must be ensured; they are necessary for equality in patient-provider relationships. Dehumanization often occurs in such situations as a person's involuntary commitment to a psychiatric institution, where the patient is stripped of her or his identity and denied all freedom and choice. The vast difference in status and power produced by physician expertise and patient dependence contributes to dehumanized care. When the patient's sex, class, or race further increases this difference, inequality is intensified. Fifth, regardless of their educational level, patients must have the right to be fully informed and to participate in decisions about their care. Sixth, practitioners must strive to achieve empathy, the ability to see the patient's point of view; this enhances understanding as well as humane care. Although physicians cannot be expected to suffer along with each patient, it is also true that a physician's indifference has an adverse effect on patients. Howard suggests that the Hippocratic ideal of the detached physician may be more applicable to interprofessional relations than to care of the sick.

Attitudes can't be changed by legislative mandate. However, the Dellums Bill offers the possibility of bringing about attitudinal change, through its recruitment policies. Since physicians would be salaried, and medical school admissions would emphasize health-work experience and encourage the recruitment of students from the populations they would serve, individuals more interested in healing than in profit might be attracted in larger numbers to medicine. Ideally, this student population would include larger numbers of women and minority members. If, in addition, medical training took place in an environment that did not rob students and other health workers of their initial idealism and enthusiasm, and if the caring aspect of medicine was stressed and rewarded, there might be a corresponding change in attitude in the medical profession.

The pros and cons of the Dellums Bill could be argued endlessly. Even if the bill isn't enacted in the near future, it does serve the purpose of stimulating debate on health care and increasing public awareness of possible options and alternatives to the present system. Vested-interest groups can be expected to resist change and oppose a medical plan that shifts control from providers to consumers. If the United States, therefore, is to have a class-free, consumer-controlled national health care system, the impetus for change will have to come from consumers themselves.

The Women's Health Movement

The women's health movement in the United States, an outgrowth of women's liberation, began to organize in the late 1960s in response to women's growing concern and dissatisfaction with authoritarian, male-dominated obstetrics and gynecology. In the intervening years, the women's health movement has demonstrated that, despite the enormous power and influence of medicine, women can challenge institutional practices and, if sufficiently dissatisfied, will create their own alternatives. The movement is both a model for consumer action and a resource for those seeking to change their health care.

In *The Women's Health Movement: Feminist Alternatives to Medical Control,*[9] Sheryl Burt Ruzek traces the history of the women's health movement. Her landmark book succeeds magnificently in demonstrating that health care is indeed a political issue. Central to the concern of feminist health activists, Ruzek explains, is "women's right to choose and decide about their own care . . . Women emphasize the need for humane practitioners working in settings that allow women to retain their life values, especially those related to autonomy."[10] Ruzek outlines five movement strategies for improving women's health care: (1) educating the public in order to close the gap in knowledge between patient and practitioner; (2) challenging physicians' exclusive license to provide certain services; (3) reducing medical professionals' control and monopoly over health-related necessities, both goods and services; (4) tailoring the size of the medical profession to fit the size of its clientele; (5) unifying medical consumers into a collective.[11]

The principal goal of the women's health movement is to restructure the content and delivery of routine care for well women — an important aspect of women's health disdained by many obstetrician-gynecologists yet under their control — and in doing so to deinstitutionalize medical authority and transform the relationship between patients and practitioners. This would help enable women to judge the quality of the care they receive, assert their rights, act decisively, and seek alternatives as desired.

Closing the Gap in Women's Health Knowledge

A successful challenge to medical authority requires a redistribution of medical knowledge from the exclusive domain of certified experts to patients themselves. Consciousness-raising groups and self-help health courses have been organized throughout the United States to teach women about their bodies, the reproductive process, and general health. Women are taught to monitor their health with breast and cervical self-examinations. Numerous publications supplement these educational efforts. *Our Bodies, Ourselves,*[12] by the Boston Women's Health Book Collective, for instance, has become a classic reference for women of all ages. Other books, newsletters, newspapers, and films informing women about health issues abound. (See the lists of resources, pages 269–274.) Efforts have also been directed at raising physicians' consciousness. For example, one feminist group in North Carolina teaches medical students to perform nonabusive pelvic examinations by demonstrating the technique on themselves and thus saving women who are unaware that they are being used as teaching material from an uncomfortable experience.

Some feminists have opted to eliminate their dependence on male physicians, preferring self-care clinics, where routine care for well women is shifted from professional experts to the women themselves. As Ruzek explains:

> Self-care clinics challenge the whole medical-professional model, in which the physician is assumed to be the only person who is competent to evaluate medical needs, propose or prescribe specific regimens or treatments and

judge the competence of other practitioners. Radical-feminist settings not only challenge these assumptions but shatter many myths about workable patient and professional roles.[13]

Health Politics

The women's health movement has taken an active role in influencing health legislation and public policy and in pressing for enforcement of existing laws and regulations through legal action. The National Women's Health Network, a nonprofit organization representing a coalition of local women's health groups, projects, clinics, health professionals and consumers, identified key health issues at a 1976 meeting, issues such as unnecessary obstetrical intervention and gynecological surgery, the federal role in health care, rape, and wife abuse, occupational health and safety, and the effective use of women as health care providers.[14]

During 1978, the Network was prominent in lobbying efforts against the Upjohn Company's attempt to secure Food and Drug Administration approval for Depo-Provera, an injectable, long-term contraceptive for women that the Network argues is a known carcinogen and that is currently marketed in Third World countries with an estimated three to five million users.[15] The organization also has mounted efforts to retain abortion as part of the inalienable right of every woman to control her body, and has opposed the elimination of public funds to finance abortions for low-income women. Public testimony has been directed at redefining contraceptive research priorities from hormones, drugs, and invasive devices, such as hormone-releasing IUDs, to mechanical or barrier methods, such as the diaphragm and cervical cap, and has also included efforts to strengthen and implement strict enforcement of proposed legislation to regulate sterilization abuse. In addition, alerts have been issued on the need for danger warnings to pregnant women about alcoholic beverages and for informed consent in the use of estrogen replacement therapy (ERT).

Because physicians do not adequately regulate themselves, feminist health activists have organized lay referral systems and patient advocate programs. In many communities women have produced health service directories that provide information on availability and cost of local services. Feminist groups have organized programs in which advocates are available to accompany women to gynecological examinations, knowing, as women do, that it is difficult for anyone "stripped and draped" to assert her rights.

Individual Solutions to Collective Problems: Protect Yourself and Work Together

Through education and the resources offered by the women's health movement, every woman can effect some improvement in her health care. Unnecessary obstetrical intervention and unnecessary surgery remain thorny problems whose solutions will require external controls over the medical profession and the reordering of health care delivery, but women who are well informed have greater control over their health when faced with a decision about obstetrical care or surgery than uninformed women.

1. Before a woman engages an obstetrician's services, she should determine the physician's attitudes toward induced labor, fetal monitoring, birth position, use of medication, anesthesia and forceps, Lamaze and advocates in the delivery room, LeBoyer technique, episiotomy, breast-feeding, and lying-in. Certain types of childbirth arrangements — for example, Lamaze, midwife-conducted birth, and home birth — eschew obstetrical intervention and will provide a natural experience if possible. Since cesarean section rates vary significantly from one hospital to another, a woman should find out whether the operation is widespread in the hospital her doctor is affiliated with.

2. A physician's recommendation for surgery should always be questioned and checked. Before a woman signs a consent form, she should make the surgeon give her a full explanation

of the surgery in plain language, including reasons for the surgery, the exact procedures to be used, the extent of the surgery (which organs will be removed), alternatives to the surgery, recuperation time, and possible risks and complications of the operation.

3. Unless there is an emergency, like an ectopic pregnancy, a second surgical opinion should be obtained. It is important to choose a second surgeon who will not profit either directly or indirectly from the surgery. The likelihood of getting a disinterested opinion is increased if the second consultation is with a surgeon not connected with the first physician's referral network and if the second surgeon understands that his or her advice is sought only as a second opinion. (This is still not adequate protection against unnecessary surgery. Second opinions are expensive and, though the government and some insurance plans may pay for them, they are beyond the means of many. Moreover, they add to the profits of surgeons and to health care costs and are another way in which consumers are victimized by the medical profession's lack of regulation.)

Our Bodies, Ourselves lists the following indications that a hysterectomy is needed:

> a) A local malignancy of the cervix or in the lining of the uterus itself.
> b) Symptomatic nonmalignant conditions — for example, an excessive number of very large fibroids on the inside of the uterus.
> c) Excessive bleeding that does not respond to hormone treatment or to D & Cs, or in cases for which these treatments may not be appropriate.
> d) Diseases of the tubes or ovaries that require removal of the uterus, too.
> e) Cancer of the uterus itself.
> f) Catastrophe during childbirth that requires removal of the uterus for the woman's survival.[16]

One of the major accomplishments of the women's health movement has been to make women aware that their problems are shared by others. In the final analysis, there are no satisfactory individual solutions to collective problems. The control and authority of physicians is reinforced by the lack of unity among patients and medical consumers. Without unity, medical consumers are unable to compare notes and work together for change. Though the barriers to restructuring health care are substantial, feminist health activists have shown that, by organizing, consumers can affect established medical power structures. The women's health movement offers a challenge to individuals who are willing to work to create a strong consumer organization that will have clout.

Notes

1. M. David Ermann and Richard J. Lundman, "Deviant Acts by Complex Organizations: Deviance and Social Control at the Organizational Level of Analysis," *The Sociological Quarterly*, 19 (1978), 55–67; M. David Ermann and Richard J. Lundman, eds., *Corporate and Governmental Deviance* (New York: Oxford University Press, 1978).
2. Rick J. Carlson, *The End of Medicine* (New York: John Wiley, 1975).
3. Victor Richards, "Surgical Education with Full-Paying Patients," *American Journal of Surgery*, 121 (1971), 217.
4. Ibid., p. 219.
5. In June, 1979, a 29-year-old Baltimore, Maryland, woman, mother of two children, was awarded $1.5 million damages in a malpractice suit for a total hysterectomy that she had not given her surgeon permission to perform. Reasons for the historically large settlement (that was more than the $1.2 million she sought and will be appealed) included the woman's inability to have additional children and the fact that she must now have estrogen replacement therapy (ERT) with its associated increased risk of breast cancer. Despite the high rates of unnecessary hysterectomies in the United States, this is one of the few cases of litigation for the unnecessary performance of the operation and demonstrates that at least one jury places a high value on women's reproductive organs.
6. Robert M. Sade, "Medical Care as a Right: A Refutation," *New England Journal of Medicine*, 285 (1971), 1289.
7. "The Health Service Act, H.R. 6894," *Congressional Record*, vol. 123, no. 75 (Washington, May 4, 1977); "The United States Health Service, H.R. 11879," *Congressional Record*, vol. 124, no. 47 (Washington, April 6, 1978).

8. Jan Howard, "Humanization and Dehumanization of Health Care," in Jan Howard and Anselm Strauss, eds. *Humanizing Health Care* (New York: John Wiley, 1975).
9. Sheryl Burt Ruzek, *The Women's Health Movement: Feminist Alternatives to Medical Control* (New York: Praeger Publishers, 1978).
10. Ibid., p. 104.
11. Ibid., p. 144.
12. Boston Women's Health Book Collective, *Our Bodies, Ourselves* (New York: Simon & Schuster, 1976).
13. Ruzek, *The Women's Health Movement*, p. 120.
14. Ibid., pp. 156-157.
15. National Women's Health Network, Press Release, October 23, 1978.
16. *Our Bodies, Ourselves*, p. 148.

Glossary of Medical Terms

Glossary of Medical Terms

Abdominal Hysterectomy: Removal of the uterus through an incision in the abdomen.

Abortion: Termination of a pregnancy. Common techniques, and the periods of pregnancy during which they are done, include vacuum suction or vacuum curettage, from 7 to 12 weeks, in which a tube is passed through the cervix into the uterus and fetal tissue is suctioned from the uterine wall; dilation and curettage, from 8 to 12 or 15 weeks, a standard gynecological procedure in which the cervix is dilated and fetal tissue removed by instrument; saline or prostaglandin, 16 to 24 weeks, in which labor is induced by the injection of an abortion-causing solution into the amniotic sac.

Amenorrhea: Absence of menstruation. May be symptomatic of a disorder if it occurs during the woman's fertile years.

American College of Obstetricians and Gynecologists (ACOG): Professional organization for obstetricians and gynecologists.

American Medical Association (AMA): Professional organization for physicians.

Amniotic Sac: Sac or bag containing amniotic fluid in which the fetus floats during pregnancy.

Anus: Opening of the rectum or large intestine to the outside.

Apgar Score: System of scoring an infant's condition one minute after birth. Impressions of heart rate, respiration, muscle tone, color, and response to stimuli are scored 0, 1, or 2. The maximum, best score is 10. The person who delivers the infant usually assigns the Apgar score.

Arrested Labor: Failure of labor to proceed through normal stages.

Attendings, Attending Physicians, Attending Staff: Physicians who have completed their medical training and may be in private practice or on the staff of a hospital.

Castration — Female: Removal of the ovaries: an ovariectomy, ovariotomy, or oophorectomy.

Cephalopelvic Disproportion: A pelvis too small for the fetal head.

Cervical Block: Regional anesthesia that blocks the pain involved in labor and delivery.

Cervix: The base or neck of the uterus through which fetus and menstrual flow pass.

Cesarean Hysterectomy: Removal of the uterus after the fetus has been taken out.

Cesarean Section: Surgical removal of the fetus by means of an incision into the uterus, usually through the abdomen.

Chief, Chief Resident: Usually a resident in senior year of training assigned responsibility for overseeing a particular service or group of interns and residents.

Clinic Patient (same as Institutional Patient): A person who obtains medical services through a clinic rather than from a private physician. May be charged a fee.

Clitoridectomy: Surgical removal of the clitoris.

Clitoris: Most sensitive spot in the genital area. It is erectile tissue that swells during sexual arousal.

Diethylstilbestrol (DES): A synthetic estrogen prescribed during the first trimester of pregnancy to prevent miscarriage up to 1970. Though the drug does not prevent miscarriage, it is linked to vaginal cancer in the female children of women who took it. It is now prescribed to prevent pregnancy as the morning after pill and should be avoided in any form.

Dilation and Curettage (D & C): A procedure to open the cervix and scrape away the lining of the uterus with an instrument called a curette. Used in abortion, diagnosis, and to treat abnormal uterine bleeding.

Dysmenorrhea: Painful menstruation; cramps.

Dysplasia: Abnormal development or changes in tissue.

Eclampsia: A major toxemia of pregnancy, accompanied by high blood pressure, convulsions, and coma. May occur during pregnancy or shortly after delivery.

Ectopic Pregnancy: Implantation of the fertilized ovum in a site other than the uterus, most frequently in a Fallopian tube, though it can also occur in the abdomen, ovary, or cervix. May cause pain.

Effacement: Thinning of the cervix prior to delivery. Measured by percentage. Ninety percent effaced means the neck of the uterus is almost completely thinned out.

Elective Surgery: A procedure that does not require immediate or emergency action. Sometimes requested by patient.

Endometrium: The mucous membrane lining the inner surface of the uterus.

Episiotomy: An incision in the perineum, the area between the vagina and the anus, to enlarge the opening through which the baby passes. Routinely performed by obstetricians in the United States.

Estrogen Replacement Therapy (ERT): Estrogen prescribed to relieve menopausal symptoms and now linked to endometrial cancer.

Fallopian Tube: The tube or duct extending from the uterus to the ovary. (There are two Fallopian tubes, one connected to each ovary.) It conveys the ovum from the ovary to the uterus and sperm from the uterus toward the ovary.

False Labor: Uterine contractions coming before the onset of actual labor.

Family Practice Physician: Specialist who has completed a residency in family medicine and is able to provide basic comprehensive primary care to persons of any age.

Fascia: The fibrous tissue covering, supporting, and separating muscles.

Fee for Service: Type of physician reimbursement in which services are paid for as they are delivered.

Fellow: At Elite and Mass, a physician who is doing additional specialized training after completing residency.

Fetal and Maternal Medicine: Care of complicated pregnancy, labor, and delivery.

Fetal Distress: The too-rapid, too-slow, or irregular fetal heartbeat; measured by fetal monitoring equipment.

Fetal Monitor: A machine that electronically records the fetal heart rate during labor. There are two basic types: external, in which electrodes are applied externally, and internal, in which electrodes are passed through the vagina and attached to the fetus's presenting part, usually the head.

Fibroid: A tumor in the uterus. Depending on size, number, and symptomology, may be removed by hysterectomy.

Flex Examination: Standard written examination required for medical licensing.

Forceps — Obstetrical: Instrument used to facilitate the delivery of a fetus. Low, mid, and high forceps refer to the position of the fetal head when the forceps are applied. High forceps are never indicated in modern obstetrics.

Grand Rounds: Meeting in which physicians and other medical personnel discuss cases and other topics of medical interest.

Gravida: A pregnant woman. Term used by obstetricians to indicate the number of times a woman has been pregnant. Gravida 3 refers to a woman who has had three pregnancies.

Gynecologic Endocrinology, Reproductive Endocrinology: Science of the development and functioning of the female reproductive organs.

Gynecologic Oncology: Diagnosis and management of female pelvic tumors.

Gynecology (gyn): The study, diagnosis, and treatment of conditions specific to women, especially those related to the reproductive organs.

Health Maintenance Organization: A prepaid health plan.

House Staff: The interns and residents of a hospital.

Hymen: A thin membrane surrounding and partly blocking the vaginal opening.

Hysterectomy: Surgical removal of the uterus, either abdominally, through an incision in the abdomen, or vaginally, through the vagina. Vaginal hysterectomies leave no scar but have a higher risk of complication. In contrast to a total, in a partial hysterectomy the cervix is left in place.

Iatrogenesis: The word coined to mean damage caused by intervention of the medical care system. Often unanticipated, such damage includes infections, overmedication, removal of healthy organs, and diagnosis and treatment of diseases that don't exist. For example, fetal monitoring may cause iatrogenic illness.

Induction of Labor: Use of oxytocin (Pitocin is one proprietary name of the drug) to stimulate uterine contractions before they normally would occur in childbirth.

Institutional Patient: See Clinic Patient.

Intern: A physician-in-training. Usually a recent medical school graduate who is receiving a year of postgraduate training before being licensed to practice medicine.

Inversion of the Uterus: A rare obstetrical complication of three types: early, in which the fundus (body of the uterus) is inverted to some degree; incomplete, in which the fundus turns inside out, protruding through the cervix but remaining within the vagina; complete, in which the uterus is completely inverted and lies entirely outside the vagina. Inversions may occur either before or after separation of the placenta.

Junior Resident: A physician in the early year or years of residency.

Labor (divided into three stages): First-stage labor begins with the earliest contractions and lasts until the cervix is dilated 10 centimeters. Transition is the period between 8 and 10 centimeters of dilation. Second-stage labor begins when the cervix is completely dilated and the baby's presenting part moves into the birth canal; it ends when the baby is born. Third-stage labor involves delivery of the placenta and takes only a few minutes.

Lamaze Childbirth: A method of prepared childbirth in which prelearned controlled breathing counteracts some of the pain of labor contractions.

Laparoscopy: A procedure used to view the inside of the abdomen through a long narrow tube (the laparoscope) inserted through a small incision. It is used for diagnostic purposes and is also a method of sterilization.

LeFort Operation: Procedure in which the vagina is surgically sewn closed. Used to treat prolapse of the uterus.

Lithotomy Position: Common, antigravitational position for childbirth in the United States; the woman lies with her back flat and thighs flexed on the abdomen.

Mastectomy: Surgical removal of the breast. Simple — removal of entire breast tissue but with pectoral muscles left intact. Radical — removal of entire breast, entire pectoral muscle, and lymph nodes in the armpit. Modified radical — removal of less muscle and retention of some nodes. Partial — removal of lump and surrounding tissue.

Menorrhagia: Excessive bleeding at the time of menstrual period, either because of a large number of days, amount of blood, or both.

Morbidity: State of being diseased; the number of sick or diseased persons in relation to a specific population.

Neonatal: Pertaining to the first four weeks after birth.

Nurse-Midwife: A nurse who has completed additional training in obstetrics and is qualified to attend normal pregnancies and deliveries.

Nurse-Practitioner (ob-gyn): A nurse who has completed additional training in obstetrics and gynecology and is qualified to provide routine and well care.

Obstetrics (ob): Branch of medicine concerned with women during pregnancy and childbirth.

Os: Opening of the cervix into the uterus.

Ovariectomy, Oophorectomy: Surgical removal of one ovary or both ovaries.

Ovary: One of a pair of organs about the size and shape of almonds located on either side of and somewhat behind the uterus. Its functions are production of reproductive or germ cells (eggs, or ova) and production of the female hormone estrogen. The corpus luteum, which forms in a follicle of the ovary after an ovum has been released, produces the hormone progesterone.

Ovum (egg): Female reproductive or germ cell.

Oxytocin: A pituitary hormone that stimulates the uterus to contract.

Pap Smear, Papanicolaou Smear or Test: Tissue is scraped from the cervix and tested for cancer and other abnormal conditions. Results are graded as follows: Class 1, clear; class 2, inflammation, irritation, infection, or mild dysplasia; class 3, borderline dysplasia, abnormal nonmalignant or premalignant cell growth; class 4, highly suspicious for malignancy; class 5, positive for malignancy.

Parity: Refers to the number of children a woman has delivered. For example, para 2 refers to a woman who has delivered two babies.

Parturition: The act of giving birth; childbirth.

Pathology: Study of the nature and cause of disease; condition produced by disease.

Pediatrics: Branch of medicine concerned with children and the diseases of childhood.

Pelvic Examination: An examination that usually includes inspection of external genitalia, insertion of a speculum, inspection of the cervix, taking of a Pap smear, palpation of uterus and ovaries, and sometimes a rectal examination. Done during labor by doctor or midwife by inserting two fingers into the vagina to evaluate pelvic dimensions, the dilation and effacement of the cervix, and the fetal presenting part.

Pelvic Inflammatory Disease (PID): A group of several pelvic infections that can affect the uterus, the tubes, or the tubes and ovaries. It can be caused by gonorrhea, certain bacteria, or specific viruses. Symptoms include pelvic pain, increasing pain with intercourse or menstruation, irregular bleeding, and chills and fever.

Pelvimetry: Measurement of the pelvis to determine whether the fetus will be able to pass through the birth canal. Done by x ray or manually.

Perineum: In the female, the area between the vulva and the anus.

Peritoneoscope: Long slender telescopic device with a light at one end and an eye piece at the other. Used to inspect the peritoneal cavity through a small incision in the abdominal wall.

Peritoneum: The membrane that lines the abdominal cavity.

Pessary: A device inserted into the vagina to function as a supportive structure for the uterus. Used for prolapse of the uterus when surgery is counterindicated.

PID: See Pelvic Inflammatory Disease.

Pitocin: One of the synthetic forms of oxytocin, used to induce or accelerate labor. It is a brand name.

Placenta: An oval spongy structure in the uterus through which the fetus derives nourishment.

Placenta Previa: Placenta preceding fetus at birth because it was implanted in the lower segment of the uterus. Usually indicates need for a cesarean section.

Postnatal: Happening after birth.

Postpartum: After childbirth.

Pre-eclampsia: A toxemia of pregnancy characterized by high blood pressure, headaches, and swelling of the lower extremities. If neglected can become true eclampsia.

Prenatal Care: Periodic examination of pregnant women to determine blood pressure, weight, changes in the chemistry of the urine, changes in the size of the uterus, and the condition of the fetus, as evidenced by heart tones and position.

Primigravida: A woman during her first pregnancy.
Primipara: A woman who is giving birth to her first child.
Private Patient: A person who receives medical care from a physician rather than in a clinic.
Prolapsed Cord: Expulsion of the umbilical cord prematurely during pregnancy.
Prolapse of the Uterus: Downward slipping of the uterus described in three degrees depending upon severity: first degree, cervix is within the vaginal opening; second degree, cervix is near the opening; third degree, cervix protrudes from the vaginal opening.
Prostaglandins: A group of fatty acid derivatives present in many tissues. Among other effects, they cause the uterus to contract and are used in second-trimester abortion.
Puerperal Fever (Childbed Fever): An infection in the reproductive tract incurred immediately after childbirth.
Puerperium: The period from delivery of the placenta until return of the reproductive organs to their normal nonpregnant state; it generally lasts from 6 to 8 weeks.
Radical Surgery: Surgery that seeks an absolute cure rather than relief of symptoms. As used at Elite and Mass, radical surgery was usually for extensive cancer, often involving tissue and organs surrounding the reproductive organs.
Resident: A physician-in-training who is taking additional clinical training after medical school in a specialized area of medicine.
Retractor: Instrument used for holding back the margins of an incision or wound.
Rounds (ward): Physicians' periodic visits to hospital patients.
Ruptured Membrane: Rupture of the amniotic sac (bag of waters) either naturally, as the result of dilation of the cervix during labor, or artificially, by instrument.
Salpingectomy: Surgical removal of one Fallopian tube or both.
Salpingo-Oophorectomy: Surgical removal of an ovary and Fallopian tube. Bilateral salpingo-oophorectomy is the removal of both ovaries and both tubes.
Senior Resident: A resident in final stages of training.
Sickle Cell Anemia: A form of anemia, found among people of African and Mediterranean descent, in which oxygen in the blood is reduced by the deformation of the red blood cells, which look like sickles.
Speculum: Instrument inserted into the vagina to permit examination of the cervix.
Spontaneous Abortion (Miscarriage): Noninduced termination of pregnancy.
Stillbirth: Birth of a dead fetus.
Stress Incontinence: Loss of small amounts of urine when there is a

sudden increase in abdominal pressure, for example from coughing, sneezing, or laughing.

Superspecialty: In obstetrics and gynecology, subfields of gynecologic endocrinology and infertility, gynecologic oncology, and fetal and maternal medicine.

Total Hysterectomy: Surgical removal of the uterus and cervix but not the Fallopian tubes or ovaries.

Tubal Ligation: Method of permanent sterilization in which a piece of each Fallopian tube is cut out and the two ends are tied off and folded back into the surrounding tissue. Can be done by an incision in the abdomen (most common postpartum procedure) or by endoscopy, in which a tube with mirrors and lights is inserted and the Fallopian tubes are visually located and then cauterized with a small instrument.

Ultrasound: Equipment that produces an image or outline of an organ, tissue, or fetus by use of inaudible sound. Used diagnostically in obstetrics.

Ureter: One of two tubes that carry urine from the kidneys to the bladder.

Uterus: Commonly called the womb, it consists of the body or upper portion (also called the fundus), the constricted central area, and the cervix. The uterus is the organ that contains the embryo and fetus from the time the fertilized egg is implanted to the time of birth. Nourishment passes to the fetus through the placenta.

Vagina: Canal that connects the vulva with the uterus.

Vaginal Hysterectomy: Surgical removal of the uterus through the vagina.

Vesicovaginal Fistula: Abnormal opening or tear in the wall between the vagina and bladder, resulting in a constant seepage of urine from the vagina. May be congenital or due to obstetrical injury or disease.

Vulva: Outer genitals, including the labia majora, labia minora, clitoris, and vestibule of the vagina.

Vulvectomy: Surgical removal of the vulva.

Work-up: Part of diagnostic process, taking patient's history and ordering tests.

Resources

Resources

Recommended Books on Women, Health, and Politics

Arms, Suzanne. *Immaculate Deception: A New Look at Women and Childbirth.* Boston: Houghton Mifflin, 1975.

Boston Women's Health Book Collective, *Our Bodies, Ourselves* (2nd ed.) New York: Simon and Schuster, 1976.

Campbell, Margaret. *Why Would a Girl Go Into Medicine?* Old Westbury, New York: The Feminist Press, 1973.

Corea, Gena. *The Hidden Malpractice: How American Medicine Mistreats Women.* New York: Jove, 1977.

Cowan, Belita. *Women's Health Care.* Ann Arbor, Michigan: Anshen Publishing, 1979.

———. *Women's Health Care: Resources, Writings, Bibliographies.* Write Belita Cowan, National Women's Health Network, 2025 I Street, N.W., Suite 105, Washington, D.C. 20006.

Dreifus, Claudia, ed., *Seizing Our Bodies: The Politics of Women's Health.* New York: Vintage Books, 1977.

Ehrenreich, Barbara, and John Ehrenreich. *The American Health Empire: Power, Profits and Politics.* New York: Vintage Books, 1971.

Ehrenreich, Barbara, and Deirdre English. *Complaints and Disorders: The Sexual Politics of Sickness.* Glass Mountain Pamphlet, no. 2, Old Westbury, New York: The Feminist Press, 1973.

———. *For Her Own Good: 150 Years of the Expert's Advice to Women.* New York: Anchor Press/Doubleday, 1978.

———. *Witches, Midwives, and Nurses: A History of Women Healers.* Glass Mountain Pamphlet, no. 1, Old Westbury, New York: The Feminist Press, 1972.

Frankfort, Ellen. *Vaginal Politics.* New York: Quadrangle Books, 1972.

Gordon, Linda. *Woman's Body, Woman's Right: A Social History of Birth Control In America.* New York: Penguin Books, 1977.

Haire, Doris. *The Cultural Warping of Childbirth.* Rochester, New York: International Childbirth Education Association, 1972.

Ruzek, Sheryl Burt. *The Women's Health Movement: Feminist Alternatives to Medical Control.* New York: Praeger Publishers, 1978.

———. *Women and Health Care: A Bibliography.* Write Program on Women, Northwestern University, 619 Emerson Street, Evanston, Illinois 60201.

Seaman, Barbara. *Free and Female.* New York: Coward, McCann & Geoghegan, 1972.

———. *The Doctor's Case Against the Pill.* New York: Avon, 1969.

Seaman, Barbara, and Gideon Seaman. *Women and the Crisis in Sex Hormones.* New York: Coward, McCann & Geoghegan, 1972. (Paperback edition, New York: Bantam Books, 1978.)

Weideger, Paula. *Menstruation & Menopause: The Physiology and Psychology, the Myth and the Reality.* New York: Alfred Knopf, 1976.

Wertz, Richard, and Dorothy Wertz. *Lying-In: A History of Childbirth in America.* New York: The Free Press, 1977.

Women's Health Newsletters and Periodicals

Boston Women's Health Book Collective, Inc., Health Packets, Box 192, West Somerville, Massachusetts 02144.

Coalition for the Medical Rights of Women News, 4079A 24th Street, San Francisco, California 94114.

Family Planning Perspectives, Planned Parenthood-World Population, The Alan Guttmacher Institute, 515 Madison Avenue, New York, New York 10022.

Health/Pac Bulletin, Health Policy Advisory Center, 17 Murray Street, New York, New York 10007.

Health Resource Guides, National Women's Health Network, 2025 I Street, N.W., Suite 105, Washington, D.C. 20006.

HealthRight, Women's Health Forum, 175 Fifth Avenue, New York, New York 10010.

ICEA News, International Childbirth Education Association, P.O. Box 20852, Milwaukee, Wisconsin 53220.

Majority Report, 74 Grove Street, New York, New York 10014.

The Monthly Extract, New Moon Communications, Box 3488 Ridgeway Station, Stamford, Connecticut 06905.

NARAL Newsletter, 706 Seventh Street, S.E., Washington, D.C. 20003.

Network News, National Women's Health Network, 2025 I Street, N.W., Suite 105, Washington, D.C. 20006.

Off Our Backs, 1724 Twentieth Street, N.W., Washington, D.C. 20005.

Quest, a Feminist Quarterly, 2000 P Street, N.W., Washington, D.C. 20009.
Women & Health, Issues in Women's Health Care, SUNY/College at Old Westbury, Old Westbury, New York 11568.
WONAAC Newsletter, Women's National Abortion Action Coalition, 150 Fifth Avenue, Room 315, New York, New York 10011.
Women's Occupational Health Resource Center, American Health Foundation, 320 East 43 Street, New York, New York 10017.

Films on Women's Health

Taking Our Bodies Back: The Women's Health Movement, Cambridge Documentary Films, Inc. P.O. Box 385, Cambridge, Massachusetts 02139.
It Happens to Us (abortion), New Day Films, P.O. Box 315, Franklin Lakes, New Jersey 07417.
Self Health, Multi Media Resource Center, 540 Powell Street, San Francisco, California 94108.

Women's Health Organizations

American Foundation for Maternal and Child Health
30 Beekman Place
New York, New York 10022

Boston Women's Health Book Collective
P.O. Box 192
West Somerville, Massachusetts 02144
(Write and they will supply information about a women's health group in your area.)

Coalition for the Medical Rights of Women
4079A 24th Street
San Francisco, California 94114

Health Research Group
2000 P Street, N.W.
Washington, D.C. 20036

International Childbirth Education Association
Box 1900
New York, New York 10001

National Abortion Rights Action League (NARAL)
250 West 57th Street
New York, New York 10019

National Women's Health Network
2025 I Street, N.W., Suite 105
Washington, D.C. 20006

Women's Health Action Movement (WHAM)
175 Fifth Avenue, Room 1319, New York, New York 10010

Women's Health Forum
175 Fifth Avenue
New York, New York 10010

Vancouver Women's Health Collective
1520 West 6th Avenue, Vancouver
British Columbia, Canada

Index

Index